THE NEW Aspirin *Alternative*

The Natural Way to Overcome
Chronic Pain, Reduce Inflammation and
Enhance the Healing Response

❖ Escape toxic prescription pain drugs
❖ Capture your flexibility and rejuvenate your
ability to be active and shed years of pain

with

Systemic Oral Enzymes

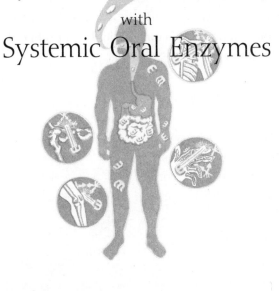

by Michael Loes, M.D., M.D.(H.)

THE NEW ASPIRIN ALTERNATIVE–*The Natural Way to Overcome Chronic Pain, Reduce Inflammation and Enhance the Healing Response* by Michael Loes, M.D., M.D.(H.)

DISCLAIMER: The material in this presentation is for informational purposes only and not intended for the treatment or diagnosis of individual disease. Please, visit a qualified medical or other health professional for specifically diagnosing any ailments mentioned or discussed in this material.

This information is presented by medical experts whose sources of information include scientific studies from the world's medical and scientific literature, doctors' patients and other clinical and anecdotal reports.

ISBN 978-1-893910-86-7

Published by Freedom Press
www.freedompressonline.com
info@freedompressonline.com
800-959-9797

Acknowledgements

There are many persons whose contributions to this book have been invaluable and to whom I would like to express our profound gratitude. First and foremost, we owe tremendous thanks to Drs. Max Wolf and Karl Ransberger, brilliant scientists and doctors who have pioneered modern systemic oral enzyme therapy. I also wish to thank scientist Helene Benitez who worked with Dr. Wolf to create what eventually come to be known as Wobenzym, the medicine of the future. The world is a better place with less pain and suffering as a result of their contributions.

I am also grateful to Joanne Spangler, whose secretarial and organizational skills are a constant encouragement to us and, of course, to the whole staff at the Arizona Pain Institute, Southwest Pain Management and Southwest Center for Pain.

Table of Contents

Appendixes

Introduction
Systemic Oral Enzymes–The Ultimate Holistic Healing Medicine

Come with me and get ready for a story that will change your life. I will tell you about a type of natural, totally safe and proven medicine called systemic oral enzymes that can help you to overcome many of the most painful maladies and conditions afflicting people today. It is like no other story that has been told before, and systemic oral enzymes are like no other medicine available anywhere in the world.

If you have ever said, "I don't want to suffer the pain of arthritis" or "I don't want to sit on the sidelines because of redness and swelling" or "I don't want to lose my ability to exercise due to muscle soreness" or "I don't know what to do about my inflammation" or "I want to reduce my risk for heart disease and cancer" or "I need help with my prostatitis, sinusitis, urinary tract infections" or "I want to do something about my aches and pains besides taking toxic pain killers," then the time is right for you to start to use systemic oral enzymes.

The miraculous healing powers of Wobenzym® N systemic oral enzymes–an underground secret healing with massive scientific documentation–are about to be unleashed in America, and, frankly, it's about time. By reading this book you will be among the first to reap the many rewards that come with regular use of the systemic oral enzyme formula that will be detailed on these pages.

What are you waiting for? If you are not yet using these miracles of nature, then you are missing out on a true fountain of life.

Enzymes are the food of the future. They excel like no other medicine or food today at strengthening the body's ability to overcome the most common injuries and chronic pain conditions.

Systemic oral enzymes are probably the greatest, virtually best kept secret in mainstream pain medicine today.

But there is only one massively proven formula in the world. It is the leading non-aspirin over-the-counter medicine in the world today, and this formula is the subject of this book.

Enzymes, the Healing Response and So Much More . . .

Enzymes are the ultimate holistic healing medicine. Besides favorably modulating your immune function and improving your overall health by lowering inflammation, you will also learn how to use systemic oral enzymes to overcome pain in many different and important chronic disease conditions.

Systemic oral enzymes can help us in so many truly important ways. I am not only going to tell you how enzymes can help you to markedly reduce important risk factors for heart disease and stroke, boost your immunity, and even prevent or reduce your risk of cancer. I will also show you how enzymes can end the pain of difficult-to-treat arthritis, lupus and other auto-immune diseases, as well as prostatitis, sinusitis, herpes, and even inflammation-related tinnitus. What is so amazing about what I am going to show you is that for each condition, there is solid, credible and often massive experimental and clinical medical validation—information that your doctor may not know about and that could mean the difference between living a life of pain or one in which you enjoy fantastic health.

Eating right with systemic oral enzymes will also likely result in loss of weight, but more importantly, your curves will improve. If you're a lady, it's likely your dress size will decrease and your complexion become soft, plush and clear, and if you are a man, you will note that angle–the one between the high part of your belt on your back and the place where you fasten that buckle in front will decrease. Getting the buckle to keep from falling south is laudable and, with systemic oral enzymes, achievable. Your pleated pants may actually begin to look like they fit. You may be able to stop considering those suspenders your wife got you last father's day.

The beauty of systemic oral enzymes is that these simple pills are such powerful and broad-spectrum biological response modifiers that at the same time you are treating chronic pain, you'll also be reducing your risk for a heart attack, stroke or cancer, and many other conditions. In the sense that enzymes have such a broad biological response within the human body and without any significant toxicity, they may work better than any of the current crop of pain relievers in use today, particularly for healing long-term chronic pain.

Unfortunately, most doctors have not yet fully understood that enzymes are absorbed, and that they do much more than just simply aid the body in digesting food.

They act inside the system, along with co-enzymes and other catalysts to modulate, enhance and restore health. This concept is not new to enzymology if doctors have been reading leading European medical journals. Unfortunately for North American pain patients, the clinical use of enzymes has been most widely practiced in Germany and its bordering neighbors, including Switzerland, Austria and Russia. Widespread use of enzymes is also being seen in Hungary, the Czech Republic, and Bulgaria. Its exposure and hence its use in the United States has been limited to topical application of wounds, and for pancreatitis. Ironically, in pancreatitis, American physicians are under the mistaken belief that giving enzymes is "resting" the pancreas by providing external replacement, when in fact, the benefit is overwhelmingly more likely attributed to the anti-inflammatory effects of enzymes on a systemic basis.

Indeed, in Germany, the systemic oral enzyme preparation detailed in this book is on record as being for many years the number one non-aspirin over-the-counter medicine for pain and inflammation and the ninth leading natural medicine among all medical drugs. We're not talking about alternative medicine. Enzymes are smart medicine and very much part of mainstream medicine elsewhere in the world.

Much like the post-its or even the first photocopiers, that at first were seen to be without a function, so also were enzymes for a long time a tool looking for a new function. Yet, now, after thousands of medical studies (virtually unknown in the United States but widely published and respected throughout the rest of the world), the proper uses for enzymes have been found. They are one of the most important natural medicines today for enhancing the healing response.

If taken on an empty stomach, they are well absorbed and get right into the battle of fighting, calming and even reversing the damage done to our body by inflammation, redness, and swelling. Over eight billion dollars is spent annually in America alone in attempts to alleviate pain and suffering related to joint tenderness and inflammation, much of this money spent on ineffective uses or unconventional treatments. We can do better. Now with systemic oral enzymes, we have the tools and the craftsmen to do so.

The Aspirin Alternative takes some recently acquired knowledge and uses it to help you get back to your God–given, genetic, optimal appearance and function.

The concept here is to utilize to the max what you ingest–to let what you ingest, get into your system where it belongs–to the cells where the catalytic energy from your mitochondria (the cellular energy factories) can be boosted. It is here where your body takes in fuel and converts it to metabolic energy.

Many–probably most of us–feel sluggish some of the time, or even most of the time. It's time to change all of that and enzymes are probably the most important daily part of your regimen that is missing. Enzymes are essential nutrients for you to put the pedal to the metal and go where you want to go at the speed you want to move.

The New Aspirin Alternative offers something else, too, that is extremely important to people who've spent months, if not years, using potentially toxic painkillers. It helps you to eliminate the debris accumulated by living. No matter whether you're married with children or single or someplace in–between, the debris of daily living accumulates quickly within your body. Having a compactor (i.e., normal digestive function) helps, but doesn't solve the problem. It just gives the appearance of helping–by making the debris look smaller. What you really need are a bunch of little helpers, energetic ones that will actually take the garbage out. Enzymes are very useful for just this. Enzymes detoxify. They are able to digest those bits of smelly, awful inflammatory garbage and turn them into something else–at least something more soluble, so that the garbage doesn't clog up your tank. Not only do enzymes break down big proteins, they also have antioxidant effects. With the right tools, cellular damage can often be zeroed out. It has been estimated that a cancer, a plaque, a hole, a clot is being formed every second of our lives. Without these defense mechanisms, such destruction would foretell our doom very quickly. Here we have yet another system acting to reduce free radical damage, and stop the aging process.

And yet the breakthrough research I will present in this book shows us that enzymes go much further. For most people who are suffering the pain of arthritis, lupus, chemotherapy, radiation, surgery and other inflammatory conditions, simply using the enzymes we educate you to use in the manner that doctors prescribe will initiate fundamental change. It may or may not be life changing, depending on what you have, to date, been doing. Most of us need all the help that we can get, however–and systemic oral enzymes are key.

I make you this promise.

Enzymes could be the gift from God that you have been seeking if you suffer from many of the most common maladies afflicting humankind. I will present true life healing stories and clinical studies supporting their use for many of the most common chronic pain conditions.

You'll not only learn how systemic oral enzymes might be the most powerful tool to date for enhancing the healing response when confronted by some of the most tragic states of disease among adults, including lupus and multiple sclerosis, but also how systemic oral enzymes can even help vulnerable children suffering childhood diabetes.

With systemic oral enzymes you'll also see the heights to which you with your fantastic health can aspire and how important systemic oral enzymes are to helping the world's most competitive, elite athletes perform at their best–even learn which Olympic Gold medallists, professional athletes and tennis champions have used systemic oral enzymes to experience the ecstasy of victory. You'll also see how systemic oral enzymes have extremely practical uses for anyone who suffers acute or chronic bronchitis, sinusitis, prostatitis, cystitis (lower urinary tract infections), and pelvic inflammatory disease. I will show their beneficial uses before and after operative dentistry, proctology and traumatology.

I will also show you how systemic oral enzymes can prevent heart disease and circulatory disorders, as well as play an important role in providing relief, if not advancing partial or total cures, for some of the most painful cases of arthritis, ulcerative colitis and Crohn's disease, multiple sclerosis, and even fibrocystic breast disease.

What We Promise

I promise that we will help you to unlock the body's own healing powers. Today's conventional pain–killer approach is changing quickly and soon to be outdated. Our goal is to help keep you in touch with all of the latest, safest and most effective breakthroughs–and also to alert you to instances when the advertising for certain drugs or nutritional supplements or other therapies is exaggerated and can either result in physical harm to you or lead you to waste your money on unproved methods.

I also know that pain relief isn't going far enough. We must not simply mask symptoms but stop degeneration and rejuvenate.

Many drugs are available to treat pain. Yet several natural agents are also equally proven to relieve pain, stimulate tissue regeneration, and, what's more, are completely safe. Unfortunately, most consumers either do not know about these substances or are unsure about their scientific validation and, therefore, hesitant to turn to them. We promise to provide you a pathway for turning on these healing powers within your own body by using one of these natural agents.

Healing is our quest. Healing the patient with pain is our focus. The Greeks used the word salubrity that brings into consciousness this seeking, an enviable state of wellness. Salubrity encompasses many of the cultural aspects of the healing arts, both modern and ancient. As we discuss pain, healing and true health, these concepts will become more and more familiar to you.

In this book, you will learn how to use enzymes to improve your health. You will learn how to eat foods for maximum bodily enzyme activity and how to detoxify your lifestyle using enzyme therapies. This book will change your life. We promise.

You can turn on the amazing healing powers in your own body and initiate dramatic improvements in your health if you are suffering from pain or risk factors for chronic diseases such as stroke, coronary artery blockages, rheumatoid arthritis,

---

The Aspirin Alternative: **About the Title**

Aspirin is a fantastic drug that relieves pain, reduces the risk of a second heart attack, and may even reduce risk of certain cancers. But, aspirin also has side effects and complications including bleeding ulcers and kidney shutdown. In fact, some experts believe that if aspirin were to have been developed today and first brought to market in the last few years (rather than more than 100 years ago) it would never be granted Food and Drug Administration approval because of these complications. Aspirin is a member of the non-steroidal anti-inflammatory drug (NSAID) family. Drug reactions from aspirin and the other NSAIDs are known to have potentially serious, sometimes fatal complications and, in fact, cause in excess of 15,000 deaths annually in America alone.

In this book it is not my intention to disparage aspirin or related NSAIDs. We have rather chosen our title metaphorically to grab your interest and say. "Here are alternatives to not only aspirin but other NSAIDs that may work equally well or better but without complications. Why not read about their massive scientific and clinical documentation and give systemic oral enzymes a try?"

osteoarthritis, or any of many other inflammatory states by following our comprehensive healing program.

You can turn on the amazing healing powers of your own body and initiate dramatic improvement in your health if you are suffering from any degenerative or destructive disease.

Yet, it should always be understood and underlined here again that you should work with your doctor. We recognize that sometimes potent complex drug therapies will be necessary to stop an acute flare-up and spare further tissue or joint destruction.

Nevertheless, I'm here to coax, persuade, and motivate you into action to get your life back on track by acting on our healing program and harnessing the amazing healing powers of systemic oral enzymes.

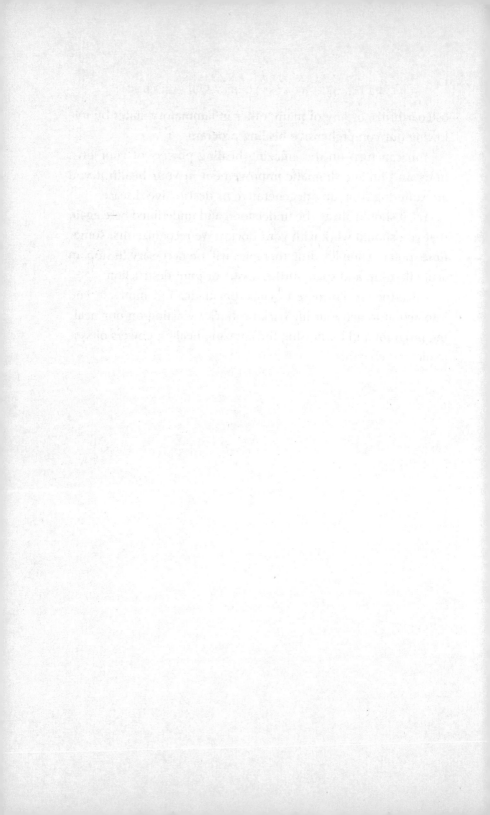

Part I

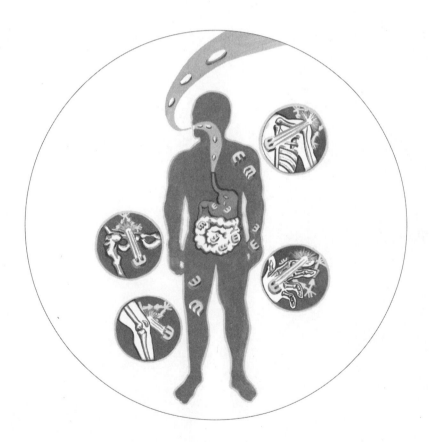

1

Not Medicine as Usual

Non-steroidal anti-inflammatory drugs (NSAIDs) are the agents most commonly used to treat pain and inflammation. This is true for osteoarthritis, rheumatoid arthritis, and for the more than one-hundred other varieties of arthritis, as well as for many other conditions, including almost all other inflammatory conditions such as sinusitis, prostatitis and cystitis, to name but a few of the more common inflammatory conditions, in which there is pain, redness, inflammation, and swelling apparent either externally (as in the case of rheumatoid arthritis) and/or within the tissues of the body (for example, as in the case of hepatitis or prostatitis).

In a sense "the cat has been let out of the bag." We know these drugs are toxic. Over 15,000 Americans per year will die from complications resulting from NSAID therapy. This is particularly true for the elderly, and for anyone with a history of peptic ulcers. In any given year, it's estimated that six percent of patients taking NSAIDs will get into serious trouble, requiring hospitalization.[1, 2]

This fact was underscored again, when bromfenac sodium (Duract) was abruptly withdrawn from the market in 1998 because of severe liver toxicity, and several associated deaths. In December 1998, the Food and Drug Administration (FDA) approved the new arthritis pain-killer, celecoxib (Celebrex), the first in a long-awaited new type of painkiller for millions of arthritis sufferers that is said to be safe on the stomach. Initial sales reports on Celebrex show it surpassed the popular sexual potency drug Viagra (i.e., sildenafil citrade) in sales during its first month. Yet, amidst all of the hype, the FDA cautioned its stomach-safe benefits may have been overplayed.[3] Celebrex will bear the same warning about side-effects as many of today's standard painkillers.

Indeed, most recently Celebrex has been linked to 10 deaths and 11 cases of gastrointestinal hemorrhage in its first three months on the market, according to a recent report in The Associated Press.[4] Half of the 10 people who died suffered from gastrointestinal bleeding or ulcers, according to reports submitted to the FDA that were obtained by The Wall Street Journal under the Freedom of Information Act. Two other deaths were attributed to heart attacks, one to drug interaction, one to a kidney disorder and one with no cause of death listed.

Another related painkiller rofecoxib (Vioxx) is just out of the gate. Huge numbers of the twenty-million arthritis patients in the United States alone have rushed to begin taking these new so-called miracle drugs.

As a medical doctor and consumer advocate, these events raise my concern to a very high level. These drugs will certainly prove to be profitable for corporate shareholders, but will they prove beneficial to the consumer? *Will their benefits ultimately outweigh their risks to you as an individual consumer?* These are questions that you must answer honestly in order to protect and enhance your health.

Typically, the healing response is *not* enhanced and the drugs employed are, to be blunt, very often, all too often, simply not in patients' best interests, in fact may be downright damaging to patients' long–term health. Your body deserves what it needs and what it craves–not what your insurance company or health maintenance organization tells you it will pay for or what your doctor, whose knowledge may be limited and even inadequate when it comes to nutritional and other complementary strategies, chooses to prescribe for you. Above all else, we are educators.

Education. It's really what being a doctor is all about. Strictly speaking, a "doctor" is a teacher. Teaching health is the best way to help patients. As one expert notes, "Teaching safe and natural healing methods is the most important missing piece in our North American health care system."[5] We doctors perform at our best–and in the true spirit of the ancient father of medicine, Hippocrates–when we *teach* patients how to stay healthy.

I'm pleased to be part of the movement that is bringing the complementary medicine message to doctors in the United States. It is my task as healers to impart what wisdom we have accumulated and to teach our patients well enough so that they may create healthy independence and freedom from potentially dangerous treatments that mask symptoms but do not stimulate the body's healing pathways.

In preparation to write this book, I reviewed the results of hundreds of clinical trials and other studies on the most common prescribed and over–the–counter drugs used throughout America and Europe. I wanted to critically examine how systemic oral enzymes, as well as other scientifically validated natural healing agents and complementary medicine strategies, compared to these other commonly used medications. I was especially careful to look for studies in which systemic oral enzymes were compared to the commonly used non-steroidal anti-inflammatory class of drugs including ibuprofen and diclofenac, as well as more powerful drugs such as methotrexate, gold salts and corticosteroids.

I wanted to know what toxicity problems were most prevalent and what you, the consumer, really need to know regarding the use of these powerful prescription and OTC drugs, which are part of the eight billion dollar pain reliever industry–in America alone.

I found while the most commonly recommended NSAIDs have some limited benefit in the short run, in the long run they simply cannot match up to systemic oral enzymes for either efficacy or safety. The NSAIDs, such as aspirin and ibuprofen, are beneficial and help to reduce swelling, heat and pain. The patient may feel better, but no rebuilding of the tissues has occurred and further degeneration may have actually occurred.

“We doctors perform at our best—and in the true spirit of the ancient father of medicine Hippocrates— when we teach patients how to stay healthy. ”

Beyond Pain

Relieving pain is an important health issue, but hopefully not the sole issue among persons whose lives are beset by chronic inflammatory disease. Relieving pain should not be confused with rebuilding and regenerating joint tissues. That is why we believe our avenues of healing are so important. In fact, patients want alternatives to NSAIDs. Dr. Benjamin Kligler, a teacher in the Beth Israel Medical Center's residency program, told the January 1999 *Physician's Financial News*, "In the last five years, doctors have become aware that patients want alternative approaches integrated into medicine. They just can't say, 'This is a lot of baloney.' People just don't buy that anymore." The information presented in this book integrates sensible and safe ways of healing inflammation and calming pain. Claims presented are backed with scientific studies, and further resources are listed so that you, the consumer and patient, can play a major part in working with your health professional and deciding what is best for you.

My goal is to help you unlock your body's own healing powers to rejuvenate your life, enabling you to feel great! Whether you suffer from arthritis, ankylosing spondylitis, backache, shingles, benign breast disease, or other forms of chronic inflammation that are draining your health and wellness, you will learn about breakthroughs in natural therapies that will help you to reclaim your life, and get you back on your pathway of super natural health and longevity.

The Difference Between Healing and Treatment

What is the difference between *treatment* and *healing*? This is a key question for anyone who truly desires great health. Treatment, in the narrowest sense, is the application of drugs or surgery, the bringing into play of some foreign object, often alien to the body's natural ecology, to stop illness' symptoms—but from the outside, usually *not* getting at the root of the problem.

Of course, emergencies, such as bacterial pneumonia, blunt force trauma, skeletal fractures and dislocations, require acute *treatment*. For the lengthening "marathon" of life today, however, we want to focus our attention on promoting healing. Healing stimulates the body's own natural powers and promotes a longer and healthier life. Your body, when all is said and done, is the greatest healing pharmacy. Turning on the healing powers of your own body is key to health.

❝Treatment *from the outside leaves the body's healing powers untapped. Healing which comes from within taps the body's own powers of regeneration.* ❞

Pain~The Epidemic

Pain, along with loneliness, is perhaps the greatest fear a human being can experience. When we are slapped with it, much like a dealt hand, we would like to fold it, but can't. The terror begins, and the search for cure or meaning ensues.

What we are looking for here is something to convert a retreat into an advance, to turn despondency into laughter and to transcend when free fall is approaching as one would envision the canoe about to go over the falls.

Pain and its closely related underlying body condition inflammation are the pairing we need to attack, to advance upon, scale and transcend. We need to understand the relationship, so as to sabotage, subterfuge, conquer, and cure.

We are a society in pain. Not all the time and not all of us. But a lot of us are in pain some, most or all of the time.

One in four Americans experience significant pain. Be it headaches, backaches, or cancer-associated pain, pain is second only to upper respiratory infections (as in the case of cold and flu) for reasons to visit a doctor.

These distressing facts tell the story:

❖ Pain causes lost days at work—a greater number on an annual basis than cancer and heart disease combined.

❖ Over 25% of American women and 14% of American men have migraine headaches–although women are three times more likely to visit a doctor for this complaint than men.

❖ Interestingly, the ratio of men to women that visit the doctor for back pain is about 1:1. More than 25 million Americans suffer chronic, disabling, painful low back pain and approximately 65 to 80 percent of the population will be afflicted with low back pain at some point during their lives.[6,7]

❖ Some 20 million Americans have arthritis, most of which is osteoarthritis, but about fifteen percent have inflammatory arthritis, including rheumatoid, psoriatic, and ankylosing spondylitis.

❖ Americans are obese, a condition that causes great psychic and physical pain. More than one–third of Americans carry greater than twenty percent excess weight, and hence suffer degenerative wear and tear on weight bearing joints, particularly the knees. Morning stiffness, activity–based grinding, and just chronic aching becomes their lot in life. The excess weight results in degenerative joint disease. Even before the X–rays, the symptoms forebode the inevitable pain.

❖ Chronic fatigue is the third most common complaint for patients seeing physicians. Pain drains and causes disruptive sleep particularly in older Americans. With loss of healthful, restful sleep, hormonal dysregulation occurs, and secondary depression.

❖ Judging from the sales of over–the–counter non–steroidal anti–inflammatory drugs (over eight billion dollars per year), we have a pill consuming society bent on drugging pain.

❖ People are increasingly reckless, population densities are greater, and cars are faster. Hence, there are more car accidents. The emergency response systems and Level I trauma units are patching up the injured better than before. But even when the structural repair seems pretty good and the orthopedic and neurosurgery doctors sign off, rehabilitation is often limited. Result: more chronic pain. Our legal system isn't helping. More pain means more gain, financial gain, that is, especially when establishing blame and damages, which often takes years.

❖ The American diet is worsening, not improving. There is more high fat, additives, and calories everywhere. Our diet is not protecting us from, but rather inflicting further, pain.

❖ Sport injuries are also taking their toll on Americans. Our pursuits are becoming more daring, more reckless, and more injury-prone.

❖ Cancer is increasing, now striking greater than one in three Americans. The pain of chemotherapy, radiation or surgery is all together too real.

What it All Means

Hopefully, these facts will alert you and not scare you. Pain can be avoided if you're lucky; it can be lessened and sometimes eliminated if you're smart. If you are not so lucky, there are potential ways to eliminate or at least manage pain enough to give you back your life so that you no longer feel strangled by it.

3
What is Pain?

Imagine arriving home after a hellish day at the office, punctuated by a scolding from your supervisor, the back-stabbing of fellow office workers, and then ninety minutes in mind-numbing rush-hour traffic–yet, without a pounding headache. Imagine a ten-hour drive to visit relatives, fighting holiday traffic, consuming terrible food, enduring boring company and, to top it all off, an awful night spent sleeping on the lumpy fold-out bed in their recreation room–and, yet, no aching back or neck. Imagine participating in strenuous physical activity all day but waking the following morning without the pain of sore joints from osteoarthritis. Imagine participating in a karate match and taking several kicks or playing in a tackle football game in your forties or even fifties but suffering no twinges or aches or pains from sport injuries. Imagine living without the bladder trauma that often occurs during childbirth or never feeling the acute pain of food poisoning from the undercooked oysters you ate the other night. Some people might think that a life without pain would be heavenly. And in some cases, it might truly be!

In fact however, life without any pain at all would be closer to hell. After all, without pain, why would a toddler yank her fingers out of the flame of a fire or off of the stove? Why would we avoid poison oak or seek help for a broken leg?

Like many dual aspects of life, pain is both good and evil. It is a complex phenomenon. We may hate it. Yet, we may need it. Its duality is maddening. And one thing we know, pain can override all other aspects of living when it becomes too intense.

No one wants unnecessary pain. But sometimes pain saves lives. A child that knew no pain would be mutilated by its own actions. An adult that knew no pain would eventually–and probably very quickly–succumb to various traumas. Pain teaches us caution. Caution keeps us alive.

And yet while pain keeps us alive, it can also keep us from living. People suffering and enduring the excruciating pain of chronic disease that lasts for days, months, years or decades, may simply wish they could die.

Pain is a robber. It takes away our joy of living. It robs us of our most precious asset: time well–spent. No matter what its cause, unmitigated pain derived from arthritis, cancer, nerve damage and other causes, both well understood and not understood at all, is the great robber of our lives. We've all lost precious time in life due to pain. Even the non–life threatening pain of a toothache, headache or facial myalgia robs us of the joy of living. And often, there are no drugs that can provide adequate relief.

Eventually pain becomes both mental and physical. There is a saying that pain is in the brain. This is insulting! It puts the blame on the victim. Think of pain as a contaminant. Pain enters our brain via the primitive hypothalamus and thalamus but eventually is transmitted to the more cerebral cortex (our mind) and becomes an overriding issue in our daily lives.

To overcome pain, it is helpful to understand pain, especially the different kinds that we experience. Of course, there is the quick and limited pain when you accidentally jab yourself with a pin. But pain can also be mental, as in the case of emotional distress caused by loss. Pain can also be a mixture of the physical and mental.

Pain often involves the release of chemical messengers known as neuropeptides. When tissue is damaged, these chemicals cause a cascade of events that affect the whole person. They are both physical and mental. Not everyone who experiences pain suffers. This may be difficult to comprehend. But, we all have different pain thresholds. Take American gymnast Kerri Strugg who hit the mat after her memorable vault at the 1996 Olympics in Atlanta, Georgia. "The whole world winced. Her pain was unmistakable," observe Mary E. O'Brien, M.D. and Donna Hoel in a recent issue of *Postgraduate Medicine*.[8] Yet, we loved her gritting her teeth, sticking out her chin, keeping a stiff upper lip and transcending. It helped, of course, that she was visualizing Olympic gold!

It's the account of the soldier who during the heat of the battle continues to fight courageously and never feels the pain of his wound and yet, once the fighting has stopped, sees blood on his boots, calls for medical attention, and faints. Or the athlete that fractured a bone but felt no pain during the heat of the competition but afterward must be injected with powerful painkillers for days, if not weeks.

We can often put pain out of mind for short periods. If other more pressing matters are on our plate, then we can forget about pain. But, eventually, pain wins out.

And, sometimes, pain persists for years. Even after the healing of an injury, phantom pain can continue. That is because pain etches its way into our nervous system, establishing pathways that never seem to die.

Doctors often speak of *nociceptive* pain–taken from the word noise for the noise receptors that fire from nerve endings when there is thermal, mechanical or chemical pain. Nociceptive pain occurs when the body's nerve fibers in the skin, bones, joints, and viscera (guts) come into contact with everyday pain culprits. For example, Fred walks into the kitchen and complains to Wilma that she has burnt dinner and reaches for the pan in the oven, which is hot.

"Yow!" shouts Fred.

Wilma scolds her husband for being an imbecile since they were having char-broiled ribs; the pain for Fred is both physical (heat) and emotional (that Wilma thinks him a dope). Fortunately, Fred has an ego the size of a woolly mammoth and Wilma's opinion will, in this case, cause Fred only momentary pain—but the burn, which is known as *thermal* pain, will persist. Another example of pain is that of a finger dislocation suffered by a martial arts practitioner (*mechanical* pain) or the aching pain after a night of drinking (*chemical*). Ideally, once the stimulus is gone, the pain should stop. But that is the ideal world—the perfect, albeit painful—world.

Acute self-limited pain is common. You get hurt and it goes away. You know just about how long a sunburn or cut finger is likely to last.

If you sprain your wrists or scrape your knee, the pain is temporary—at least, most of the time. Musculoskeletal trauma is mostly of this type. When there is a defined trauma to the body, a healthy body is able to heal rapidly.

Sometimes, pain problems come back, much like the mythological beast that the warrior has slain only to see reappear out of the grave. Such conditions usually have a medical diagnosis and are associated with pain on an intermittent basis. The most common of these are stone diseases (kidney or gall bladder) or chronic infections or degeneration, such as toothaches or deteriorating joints. Illnesses such as intermittent cystitis, pancreatitis, or porphyria will present like this. Sometimes, and only sometimes, is migraine truly intermittent. Often, migraine becomes chronic.

However, when these irritating signals continue chronic pain occurs. If the pain is allowed to continue, untreated, and uncorrected, the pain continues, and in fact amplifies, to more generalized areas outside the original areas receiving these signals.

The concept is known as sensitization where the pain goes central–causing changes in the brain and spinal cord. The result is that **pain generalizes** and the area that hurts gets larger. This occurrence is common, particularly after cumulative trauma, most commonly after multiple car accidents, and repetitive or sports injuries. The term "post–traumatic fibromyalgia" fits many of these individuals.

But sometimes, nerves are permanently altered. Your body may even grow new pain nerves. This causes additional pain messages to be sent via the spinal cord to the brain. That means although healing may appear to be complete, you can still be exquisitely sensitive to pain in the area of the original wound.

"Pain is not just a symptom of an injury," says Dr. Allan Basbaum, chairman of the department of anatomy at UC San Francisco. "Under some conditions, it's really a disease of the nervous system."

In other words, the injured pain nerves may go through changes that initiate long–term pain–related problems. This is especially the case in long–term pain patients. For this reason alone, it is critical that pain be treated quickly and effectively as a way of preventing long–term problems.

We do not believe that stoic acceptance of pain is acceptable. There is absolutely no reason to endure pain without attempting to relieve it. Pain persistence can lead to many long–term problems. These can be emotional, mental, even social, impairing both intimate and casual relationships. Pain, left untreated, can color all aspects of life. And, apparently, many of us do leave our pain untreated. Estimates are that by the time a person in pain visits a doctor specializing in pain management they have endured that pain for seven years or more! That's a long time to live in pain. The doctor then must deal with all aspects of that pain which may infiltrate into many areas of the person's life.

We can teach people to better cope with pain. The brain is a learning organ. It attempts to accommodate. When it cannot, disruptive patterns or messages occur. This sensitization of the central nervous system causes chronic pain, which is not nociceptive in character, but has been imprinted into the memory and often the behavior of the individual. The result is chronic, non-cancer pain–the chronic pain syndrome. Although the term "chronic pain syndrome" is discouraged now favoring the diagnostic term: Pain Disorder with Psychological Factors, or Pain Disorder with Psychological and Medical Factors, the result is the same–pitiful individuals who have become victims of their painful bodies.

"When a pain's of short duration, you can cope with it," says Dennis Turk, Ph.D., a psychologist and professor of anesthesiology at the University of Washington, Seattle. "But what do you do when there's no end–when it's 365 days a year, 24 hours a day? It's no surprise that these people get depressed."

Historically, chronic pain was divided into chronic benign pain (non-malignant) and chronic progressive pain (usually cancer associated). Now, a simpler approach is usually used–chronic non-cancer pain and chronic cancer pain.

Chronic pain is very real, certainly not trivial. There may or may not be a nociceptive stimuli. In other words, there may or may not be persistent thermal, chemical, or mechanical problems, which are readily apparent from exam, lab results or X-rays, perpetuating the pain.

The treatment is to understand the patient, the primary pain problems and the co-morbidities. You must treat them all with a balanced approached.

If the object is to close as many pain gates as possible, this may lead to use of medically prescribed anti-depressants with their own witches brew of complications, thus worsening the overall health of the patient and, in a sense, leading to further depression over their dependency on these powerful, and all too frequently toxic, drugs.

Someday, we may have safe and effective drugs that can alter the pain response and prevent long-term subtle damage to the nervous system. But at present our best drug is not a drug at all but rather a natural medicine–systemic oral enzymes.

Whether the pain is "nociceptive" or not, pain is an individual experience and a healing program must be individually tailored with integrative strategies. In a nutshell, you either have acute or chronic pain. Identifying your type of pain is helpful because the treatment is likely to be different.

The Gates of Pain

We know a lot about pain, but conveying the medical or scientific information often requires a model. The model developed primarily by pain pioneers Drs. Ronald Melzack and Patrick Wall explains pain primarily by discussing various "gates."

You can open and close these gates. The nerves relaying pain information to the central nervous system use various pathways or channels. There are gates on these channels.

Below is some basic information about how to open and close gates. When it comes to pain, you would like to be able close them firmly shut.

Pain Gates: The Keys and Locks

The gate theory of pain, developed and revisited by Melzack and Wall, since 1968 continues to be widely accepted as the best tool for understanding pain, and treating it. To treat pain, you must lock the gates. Failing to lock them, or foolishly opening them leads to exacerbation of pain, and often the chronic pain syndrome.

Do the following to close the gates:

- ❖ Restful sleep.
- ❖ Think positive healing thoughts.
- ❖ Sensible exercise and regular massage.
- ❖ Specific nutritional supplements (systemic oral enzymes, glucosamine sulfate).
- ❖ Specific types of acupuncture.
- ❖ The right kind of exercise–usually general aerobics.
- ❖ Self hypnosis visualization techniques.
- ❖ Sensible weight reduction.
- ❖ Counter–irritant techniques.
- ❖ Selective dietary avoidance.
- ❖ Neuromuscular re–education.
- ❖ Specific movement therapies–FeldenKreis, Trager, Rolfing.
- ❖ Prayer.

Do not do the following; if you do, you are opening your pain gates:

- ❖ Hold on to your fear.
- ❖ Smoke, or chew tobacco.
- ❖ Drink more than two servings of wine, beer or other alcohol a day.
- ❖ Indulge in caffeine.
- ❖ Make a habit of aspartame containing beverages.
- ❖ Feast on granulated sugar.

* Eat a high animal fat diet.
* Sleep excessively.
* Exercise only on a random infrequent basis.
* Whine and pity yourself.
* Take daily over-the-counter analgesics.

The Bottom Line

* Pain is real. It can be physical or mental or both.
* Pain can be self-limiting or it can become chronic and spread throughout the body and become part of our lives, physically, mentally and emotionally.
* Pain should be treated immediately to avoid long-term nerve changes that may result in persistent pain.

4

How Pain is Usually Treated

Physicians often face a real dilemma. First, many of their patients want–indeed, demand–quick, almost instant pain relief. They come in doctor's offices and demand prescriptions they truly believe are going to prove to be magic bullets. Even though physicians know about the complications, particularly the very serious complications associated with the use of NSAIDs and their more potent cousins, the corticosteroids, they continue to prescribe these medications. This may be because very often, physicians simply don't know about other safer avenues. At other times, they simply *hope* that the complications will be minimal and, yet, provide much needed pain relief.

The key is *pain*. As healers, doctors are attuned to relieving pain.

Indeed, pain is relevant and prevalent. One in six Americans lives in pain. "No single sickness comes close to equaling pain in terms of the number of people affected," say O'Brien and Hoel. Interestingly, they also observe, "Until recently, pain management, especially chronic pain management, was seldom included in medical curricula. In fact, pain was, and still generally is, considered an essential part of the human experience. Those who bear the greatest pain are accorded the greatest respect, and courage and moral strength continue to be tied up in the ability to withstand pain."[9]

Non-steroidal Anti-inflammatory Drugs

Pain today is often usually treated with non-steroidal anti-inflammatory drugs (NSAIDs) or analgesics. Examples of NSAIDs are aspirin, diclofenac, and ibuprofen which are quickly effective against pain and relieve the most disturbing symptoms for patients (see table 4.1). Other drugs, known as analgesics, are also used for pain relief, including acetaminophen (Tylenol) which has

---

THROUGHOUT HISTORY doctors have experimented with a wide range of drugs and other procedures, some safe and not so safe, for relieving pain.[10] O'Brien and Hoel traced the history of some of the major attempts at alleviating pain in their October 1997 article in *Postgraduate Medicine*.

According to O'Brien and Hoel:

❖ Sir Christopher Wren, the 17th Century English architect and professor of astronomy at Oxford University, was perhaps the first person to successfully administer intravenous anesthetic, which he did in 1659. Dr. Wren wanted to know what the effects were of both opium and alcohol when administered together directly into the blood. In a ritual that some may call patently inhumane, he injected a dog with opium in warm sack (sherry). Predictably, the dog was stupefied and begged for more. An interesting scientific tidbit, note O'Brien and Hoel, is that Dr. Wren's experiment made anesthesiology history relatively late—not until the 19th century.

❖ In 1830, Napoleon's chief surgeon Dominique-Jean Larrey espoused carbon dioxide anesthesia to induce "suspended animation."[11]

❖ On a lighter note, the two medical researchers note that in the 1840s, doctors enjoyed spirited social lives by holding "laughing gas" parties and frolics.[12] In a sober moment, some students began to consider using the gases for more serious medical

(continued)

---

only weak anti-inflammatory properties and is not considered a true NSAID but is effective as an analgesic for mild to moderate pain. Almost all NSAIDs are orally administered with the exception of ketorolac (Toradol) which is available both by oral and pareneteral routes. Indomethacin and aspirin are available as suppositories. Only choline magnesium (Trilisate) and ibuprofen (Motrin) come in a liquid.

(continued)

issues. One such student at the University of Pennsylvania School of Medicine Crawford W. Long was a regular at these frolics. When he returned to Georgia in 1841, he held the parties himself but gradually began to notice that people seemed to not feel their bumps and bruises from these ancient, rowdy "raves." He made medical history on March 3, 1842 when he operated on a patient to remove a tumor from the neck while using ether (the patient inhaled the ether not Dr. Crawford!)[13]

❖ In 1850 James Simpson experimented with chloroform and convinced Queen Victoria to use it during childbirth.[14]

❖ In 1884 Sigmund Freud, who believed cocaine could combat morphine addiction, encouraged a colleague to use it for eye surgery.[15]

❖ In 1982, the Nobel Prize award went to scientists who figured out how aspirin worked.[16]

❖ By the 1990s, pain relief on demand had become the American way of life and quality-of-life issues superseded addiction fears.[17]

❖ Finally O'Brien and Hoel say that by 2010, techniques may allow us to supersede in the process before pain is ever recognized by the brain.[18]

2010? That's long way away when you're suffering pain *now*.

Table 4.1

Non–steroidal Anti–inflammatory Drugs (NSAIDs) Most Commonly Used for Pain Treatment

Generic Name	Trade Name	Usual Daily Dose
Aspirin	Bayer	4 to 10 grams per day
Aspirin (12 hour)	Zorprin	4 to 10 grams per day
Choline magnesium Trisalicylate	Trilisate	750 mg 2x
Diclofenac	Cataflam, Voltaren	50 mg 2x
Diclofenate potassium		50 mg 3x
Diflunisal	Dolobid	500 mg 2x
Etodolac	Dolobid, Lodine	400 mg 3x
Fenoprofen	Nalfon	600 mg 2x
Flurbiprofen	Ansaid	100 mg 3x
Ibuprofen	Advil, Motrin, Nuprin	800 mg 3x
Indomethacin	Indocin	50 mg 3x
Ketoprofen	Orudis	75 mg 3x
Ketoprofen delayed release	Oruvail	200 mg 3x
Meclofenamate	Meclomen	50 mg 3x
Mefanamic acid	Ponstel	250 mg 4x
Nabumetone	Relafen	1,000 mg 2x
Naproxen	Aleve, Anaprox	500 mg 2x
Naproxyn	Naprosyn	500 mg 2x
Oxyprozin	Daypro	1,200 mg 4x
Piroxicam	Feldene	20 mg. 4x
Salsalate	Disalcid, Salflex, Mono-Gesic	1,000 mg 2x
Sulindac	Clinoril	200 mg 2x
Tolmetin	Tolectin	400 mg 3x

NSAIDs are an important component in balanced analgesia in the management of both acute and chronic pain. NSAIDs have a direct action on spinal nociceptive processing with a relative order of potency which correlates with their capacity to inhibit the enzyme cyclo-oxygenase (also known as COX) activity. There are two isoforms of cyclo-oxygenase–COX-1 and COX-2. What's important for our purpose is that various NSAIDs inhibit the isoforms differently, and it is felt that when the COX-1/COX-2 inhibitory ratio is high, there is less gastric or kidney problems. For example, ketorolac, nabumetone and the newer agent meloxicam appear to have more favorable profiles.

There are now nearly 30 pharmaceutical agents classified as NSAIDs (Table 4.1). There are some nonsteroidal agents which have anti-inflammatory effects, yet are not usually considered traditional NSAIDs. One is colchicine which is largely effective only in acute gouty arthritis. It is not an analgesic and usually does not provide relief in other types of pain–though there is considerable experience that this agent helps when administered intravenously in low back pain syndromes. Other agents which have anti-inflammatory effects but are not thought of as nonsteroidals are methotrexate, chloroquine, penicillamine, and the gold salts. The major mechanism for these agents is immunological and although they are not steroids and do have anti-inflammatory properties, these drugs are not generally discussed in the same context.

One reason there are so many different brands is that each particular drug works a little differently with individual patients. Each of the NSAIDs has varying chemical structures and some authors have put them into different classes. Their metabolism, absorption, volume of distribution, protein binding, and elimination pathways in the body all vary according to their structure. What's more there are drug interactions and effects on the blood, which will also differ according to their structure. For example, indomethacin is a methylated indole, and sulindac, though closely related to indomethacin, is a sulfoxide. The side effects are very different. Indomethacin tends to cause fluid retention, and

NSAID Drug Interactions

Antacids–May decrease the absorption of NSAIDs.

Anticoagulants–As a group, NSAIDs are highly protein bound and when given with anticoagulants, some displacement of coumadin will occur, hence potentiating the effect of coumadin. NSAIDs also directly affect platelets; they reversibly inhibit platelet aggregation (except for aspirin where the effect is not reversible). The effect will parallel the drug elimination time. Hence, for drugs with long elimination times such as piroxicam and oxiprozin, the effect will be days. Giving NSAIDs in patients who are receiving blood thinning medication is not always contraindicated, but caution is advised! Because nonacetylated NSAIDs such as salsalate and choline magnesium salicylate do not directly affect platelet function, they may be safer, but can still potentiate coumadin by displacing protein bound drugs.

Anti-rheumatic agents–Many drugs used in rheumatoid arthritis such as azothiaprin (Immuran), penacillamine (Depen, Cuprimine), gold compounds and methotrexate, cause bone marrow toxicity, including decreases in the white blood cells and platelets. NSAIDs may potentiate their toxicity.

Corticosteroids–Patients who take corticosteroids concurrently are at higher risk for NSAID-induced gastropathy.

Diuretics–The action of diuretics may be potentiated with concurrent use of NSAIDs.

Lithium–The pharmacologic activity of lithium is heightened in patients taking NSAIDs. One proposed mechanism is decreased renal clearance because of decreased renal prostaglandin synthesis.

Oral hypoglycemia agents–Several NSAIDs (fenoprofen, naproxen and piroxicam) have been noted to potentiate oral hypoglycemic agents, primarily by displacing sulfonylureas from plasma protein binding sites.

Phenytoin (Dilantin)–The effect of phenytoin may be potentiated, again because NSAIDs have a high affinity for protein binding sites and can displace it. This effect has been shown with the same agents noted to displace sulfonylureas (fenoprofen, naproxen and piroxicam).

Probenecid (Benemid)–This agent has been shown to increase plasma levels of indomethacin, naproxen, ketoprofen, and meclofenamate. Hence, a lower dosage of these NSAIDs is advised when given with probenecid.

Adapted from Hence, P.K. and Willkens, R.F. *Patient Care* (Review), December 15, 1994

headaches; sulindac does not. Indomethacin is, however, some-how effective in the headache syndrome known as *hemicrania continua*, and sulindac is not. Some doctors advocate that if one agent doesn't work, select one from another class on the retrial. This view may not be well supported, at least as far as efficacy is concerned. If there are problematic side effects, however, then switching classes may be of value.

Most analgesics and NSAIDs can be safely used for two to three days, and many are sold as OTC drugs with reduced rec-ommended dosages. Obviously, instances occur when the use of these drugs is the best course of action. No one is calling into

Table 4.2

Comparative NSAID Toxicity Scores

Drug	*Toxicity Score* *from least toxic (1.00) to most toxic (9.00)*
Salsalate	1.00
Ibuprofen	1.25
Diclofenac	3.57
Fenoprofen	3.57
Sulindac	4.75
Naproxen	5.20
Ketoprofen	6.00
Indomethacin	6.25
Piroxicam	8.00
Tolmetin	8.73
Meclofenamate	9.00

Data based on serious reactions per million prescriptions, based on data from the Committee on Safety of Medicine, *British Medical Journal*; 1986; 292: 614 and 292: 1190–1192, 1986; Griffin, M.R., et al. *Annals of Internal Medicine*, 1991; 114: 257–263; Fries, et al. *Arthritis, Rheumatology*, 1991; 34: 1353–1360.

question their value in appropriate situations. However, using these drugs instead of and without trying our alternatives is due to lack of healing insight; although these drugs are anti-inflammatories, they do not stimulate healing.

When these drugs are used for longer periods, virtually all patients suffer some complications which can range from micro-bleeding in the gastrointestinal tract to liver or kidney toxicity. It is extremely important when using these medications to follow all label instructions and precautions. (See Table 4.2 for a listing of least to most toxic NSAIDs.)

What's more, these medications may have interactions with other drugs which you may be using. For this reason, if you are using other drugs, you should use them only if you have consulted with your physician. Also of note, people over 65, those with ulcers, smokers and especially people on cortisone-type medications may all be advised against using NSAIDs because of the greater risk for complications.

What about aspirin? One of the most commonly used OTC drugs is aspirin, which is commonly recommended for osteoarthritis. It does, in fact, relieve pain and inflammation, is inexpensive, and can also help to prevent heart attacks and stroke. But it often must be used at a very high dose, four to eight grams per day; and, at these higher doses, toxicity often occurs including tinnitus and gastric irritation. We believe it is probably better to use enterically coated aspirin, if you're going to use this pain reliever at all. Better yet, we suggest that you try our recommended alternatives, especially systemic oral enzymes, to address your rheumatoid arthritis- and osteoarthritis-related and other pain conditions.

Non-Narcotic Drugs

In more extreme cases of arthritis we may also use other more powerful pain relievers which are either injected or taken orally. These include steroids which may be taken orally, or injected directly into the joints. For example, two nonnarcotic pain relievers include ketorolac (Toradol) and tramadol (Ultram). Ketorolac, although an NSAID, is available as an injection drug and usually gives rapid, though short–acting, pain relief. Oral tramadol is available for moderate to severe pain. When introduced into the United States market in 1996 from Europe, it was classified by the FDA as a non–narcotic, and considered to have little to no potential for dependence or addiction. Yet, caution is now being advised in that some cases of addiction have been reported. Also of note, is that tramadol has been associated with seizures in susceptible individuals, especially when given at high doses. This risk increases if it is given concur-

---

Table 4.3

Narcotics Most Commonly Used for Pain

Generic Name	*Trade Name*
Codeine with acetaminophen	Tylenol #3, Phenaphen #3
Dihydrocodeine	Synalgos DC, DHC Plus
Hydrocodone with acetaminophen	Vicodin, Lorcet, Lortab
Methadone	Dolophine
Morphine sustained release	Ms Contin, Oramorph, Kadian
Oxycodone sustained release	OxyContin
Pentazocine	Talwin
Pentazocine with acetaminophen	Talacen
Propoxyphene	Darvon
Proproxyphene with acetaminophen	Darvocet
Propoxyphene with aspirin	Darvon Compound

rently with anti-depressant drugs such as desipramine (Norpramin) and doxepin (Sinequan). Caution has also been advised with agents known as selective serotonin re-uptake inhibitors including fluoxetine (Prozac), sertraline (Zoloft), and paroxetine (Paxil).

Extent of the NSAID Gastropathy Problem

The PDR Family Guide to Prescription Drugs warns about **ibuprofen** (Advil or Motrin), **indomethacin** (Indocin), **sulindac** (Clinoril) and **tolmetin sodium** (Tolectin): "You should have frequent checkups with your doctor if you take Ibuprofen [Indocin, Clinoril or Tolectin] regularly. Ulcers or internal bleeding can occur without warning."[20]

In fact, this warning applies to virtually all NSAIDs.

Because irritation to the stomach lining is so commonly associated with this broad family of drugs, some doctors may recommend that you also take misoprostol (Cytotec), a prostaglandin E1 look-alike (analog), which protects the stomach lining and decreases stomach acid. It is prescribed at 200 micrograms four times a day with food and has been effective at decreasing gastric ulcers (not duodenal ulcers) in patients on NSAIDs.

Two 12-week, randomized, double-blind trials in patients with osteoarthritis who had gastrointestinal symptoms but no ulcers were conducted.[21] These patients were using typical NSAIDs such as ibuprofen, piroxicam, and naproxen. Use of misoprostol daily significantly reduced ulcer incidence in those using the medication.

Although most of misoprostol's complications are relatively minor and include nausea, flatulence, headaches, dyspepsia, vomiting and constipation, the drug may cause abortions. It should never be given to women who are pregnant or who intend to become pregnant.[22] The *Physicians' Desk Reference* gives it, black box warning, and this is not to be taken lightly.

Although antacids and sucrafate (Carafate) are often given to patients complaining of hyperacidity, these agents have not been shown to decrease the incidence of gastric ulcers for patients on NSAIDs.

J.F. Fries and colleagues at Stanford have studied this issue in rheumatoid arthritis patients over the past ten years by coordinating information *(cont.)*

Narcotic (Opioid) Drugs

Narcotic drugs may also be used (see Table 4.3). For osteoarthritis, the most commonly used narcotics are propoxyphene (Darvon) and codeine, although oxycodone, pentazocine, and hydrocodone

---

Extent of the NSAID Gastropathy Problem (continued)

from the American Rheumatism Association Medical multi-center Information System (ARAMIS). Their results include the following:

❖ Gastrointestinal tract complications associated with NSAIDs are the most common serious adverse drug reactions in the United States

❖ NSAID-associated gastropathy can be estimated to account for at least 2,600 deaths and 20,000 hospitalizations each year in patients with rheumatoid arthritis alone.

❖ The rate of complications in patients with rheumatoid arthritis patients studied prospectively demonstrated that approximately six percent per year got into trouble with their NSAIDs, experiencing a significant gastrointestinal side effect with about 1.3 percent of patients requiring hospitalization.

❖ A large majority of these patients did not have preceding GI problems and prophylactic treatment with antacids and H2 blockers were not found to be of value.

❖ The relative risk of a GI-provoked hospitalization was more than five times greater in patients taking NSAIDs.

❖ A toxicity index showed buffered aspirin, salsalate and ibuprofen emerging as the least toxic with tolmetin sodium, meclofenamate and indomethacin as the most toxic.

❖ The most important risk factors are higher age, use of prednisone, previous NSAID GI toxicity, prior GI hospitalization, and high functional disability (based on American Rheumatology Association classification).

(*Clinical Rheumatology*, 1987; 6 Suppl. 2: 93-102; *Gastroenterology*, 1989; 96(2 Pt Suppl): 647-655; *Arthritis and Rheumatism*, 1991; 34(11): 1353-1360; *Scandinavian Journal of Rheum.*, 1992; Suppl 92: 21-24; *Journal of Rheum.*, 1995; 22(5): 995-997; *Scandinavian Journal of Rheum.*, 1996; Suppl 102: 3-8; *Archives of Internal Medicine*, 1996; 156(14): 1530-1536.)

may also be used. These may be combined with acetaminophen or aspirin. While these drugs may facilitate quick pain relief and allow for more activity during the day as well as rest or sleep in cases of truly severe pain, these are extremely powerful, often addictive medications and should be used only for short periods of time.

The preferred medical term is opiate or opioid, rather than narcotic, to avoid the connotation that these medical drugs cause one to go to sleep from the Greek word for sleep narcosis. Opiates are specifically those drugs such as morphine and codeine that are physically derived from opium. Most drugs in this family act on the opioid receptors but are semi-synthetic or synthetic; hence, these partially or totally synthesized substances are more properly called opioids, indicating that they are synthesized as opposed to being naturally derived.

For arthritis, the most commonly used drugs are propoxyphine (Darvon), codeine (Tylenol #3 and #4) and hydrocodone (Vicodin and Lorcet), although oxycodone (Percodan and Percocet), particularly the sustained released form (OxyContin), is becoming increasingly used. These agents may be combined with acetaminophen or aspirin and frequently are sold in fixed combinations. It is important to note that the amount of acetaminophen in a fixed combination may pose significant complications in that it is recommended daily intake of acetaminophen *not* exceed four grams per day. Exceeding this upper limit may cause liver or kidney problems, or both, a warning not to be taken lightly.

While these drugs may facilitate quick pain relief and allow for more activity during the day as well as rest or sleep in cases where pain disrupts rest, these drugs are powerful and are known to cause dependence and, in some cases, addiction. Dependence means that sudden cessation of the drugs will precipitate a withdrawal reaction. Addiction, on the other hand, means that some-how a preoccupation or obsession with the drug's use may occur whereby the patient develops compulsive behaviors, seeking frequent use of the drugs in spite of known harm. While the latter is uncommon, physicians are rightfully wary of using these drugs on a long-term basis. Prescribing them should be done only when conservative therapies have failed, and the patient clearly understands the risks and benefits of long-term use. Careful supervision, preferably by a pain management physician, is warranted, and it's unlikely that prescriptions will be refilled unless the patient is seen face to face by the prescribing physician.

Narcotic drugs are seeing an increased usage in advanced pain states and even more so in the severe inflammatory arthritis disorders (rheumatoid, ankylosing spondylitis, psoriatic arthritis). Most of the time, the weaker or less potent opioids are used and are formulated with either aspirin or acetaminophen. Part of this increasing usage is due to the advocacy position taken by algologists (physicians specializing in pain management), and more recently articulated by a consensus statement from the American Academy of Pain Medicine.[25] Data is abundant that functionality improves and addiction does not occur if a legitimate medical condition, cancer, or non-cancer, accompanied by severe pain, is treated aggressively, within a pain management treatment plan. While these drugs may facilitate pain relief, they are not without side effects and significant expense. The intent with opioids as with other pain medication is to enhance sensible activity, and improve rest–to restore to a reasonable level of well being. Even the stronger opioids such as morphine, methadone and sustained release oxycodone are being used. The latter, oxycodone, in fact, made it into the *Physicians' Desk Reference* with its studies for non-cancer pain. This was a first for an opioid to come out and basically say to doctors, "Look, I'm here. I can help. I have the studies to prove it."

Having said this, our position is to prevent pain and disability by early recognition and treatment, primarily with sensible diet, lifestyle changes, and opioids only in advanced disease under careful supervision. Physical dependence will occur to opioids, whether they are strong or weak, and physical withdrawal will occur, if stopped abruptly; agitation, hyperhidrosis (cold sweats), diarrhea and confusion also may occur.

There is also another class of drugs, known as mixed agonists/antagonists, which should be mentioned. They are synthetic narcotics and they are occasionally used for pain control. These drugs include:

Generic Name	Trade Name
Pentazocine	Talwin-NX, Talacen
Nalbuphine	Nubain
Butorphanol	Stadol, Stadol NS
Buprenorphine	Buprenex

Only pentazocine (Talwin-NX, Talacen) is available in oral form, and likely to be useful only in some cases of advanced arthritis. The property that these compounds have in common is that they have mixed activity on the narcotic receptors. They will enhance pain relief but only to a certain point. They are said to have a "low ceiling effect," which means that a small amount may be helpful but if the dose is increased, there are significant complications which are related to an antagonistic effect on the narcotic receptors. Worse yet, if the patient is given one of these mixed agents when already on a strong narcotic, it can precipitate persons into a withdrawal syndrome. Nalbuphine, butorphanol and buprenorphine are available only in injectable form. For the pain associated with labor and delivery, nalbuphine (Nubain) and butorphanol (Stadol) are used frequently, but they are best avoided for treating arthritis. Of note is that butorphanol also is available in a nasal spray (Stadol NS) that is being marketed primarily for migraine headaches. For arthritis, however, it is best to avoid this drug.

Cortisone Medications

The most powerful anti-inflammatory drugs are the cortisone-type medications, or corticosteroids. They may offer complete pain relief and relieve almost all swelling as well. Doctors try to eliminate their serious side effects by giving as low a dose as possible and using injections at the site of inflammation.

However, these drugs should be used only as the very last resort because of their significant long-term complications which include thinning bones (osteoporosis) and fractures, cataracts, glaucoma, high blood pressure, stomach irritation and bleeding, weight gain, frequent infections, and worsening of diabetes mellitus.

Antibiotics

Occasionally, we find antibiotics recommended for some forms of inflammatory arthritis, because of potential bacterial etiologies. The use of antibiotics can increase risk for serious yeast infection; however, their use may be indicated if natural healing pathways for supporting immune function don't seem to do the trick alone. If antibiotics are used, be sure to use a quality probiotic supplement with various friendly bacterial cultures and either inulin or fructooligosaccharides to help in recultivating the body's friendly bacteria.

Common Pain Drugs Inhibit Healing

As physician and educator, our goal is to prevent pain when we can, alleviate it when we must, and deter disability when able, by early recognition and treatment with sensible diet and lifestyle changes. Pharmaceutical agents should be reserved for progressive pathology when conservative measures have either failed, or when the emergency of a situation clearly warrants quick and powerful intervention. Modern medicine is powerful. We recognize this. Yet, an ounce of prevention is often worth a pound of cure. Are physicians willing to take the time to listen and to educate? Certainly, we believe our position of responsibility warrants such.

No doubt, these fast acting drugs relieve pain. Believe it or not, unfortunately, that is not all that they do. They inhibit the repair processes your tissues desperately require in order to effect their healing. On the other hand, our recommended agents relieve pain and set the stage for tissue or cartilage stabilization and regrowth, a potentially superior health strategy that all patients should know about.

Obviously, instances occur when the use of these drugs is the best course of action. No one is calling into question their value in appropriate situations. However, in the case of chronic pain, we call the use of these drugs instead of or without other safer pathways to be medical treatment in the most narrow sense; we repeat, it is treatment without insight because these drugs do not cure or stimulate the healing of the underlying degenerative disorder which proceeds.

Take the more than one-hundred form of arthritis, one of the commonest chronic pain states in America today. As early as 1978 researchers from Rotta Research Laboratories (Milano, Italy) reported NSAIDs actually inhibit the body's ability to produce cartilage cells. They pointed out that the metabolism of the cartilage may even be impaired and the degenerative process accelerated using these drugs. Non-steroidal anti-inflammatory agents, therefore, should be given only for a short period time, when pain is very severe, they asserted.

Researchers, writing in Current Medical Research and Opinion, noted:

"Most of [the typically prescribed drugs] have proved to reduce the metabolic capacity of the cartilage, and this could lead possibly to an impairment of articular function in the long run. Most of these preparations, moreover, cannot be administered as long as necessary, either because of inconvenience to the patient or because of severe side-effects, usually gastric."[24]

José M. Pujalte, M.D. and co-investigators concluded in the same journal that, "In this long run this could result in an even worse condition."[25]

This finding of a poorer state of overall skeletal, joint and tissue health, after the use of common arthritis drugs, has been verified in many studies published in journals such as *Lancet* and the *Journal of Bone and Joint Surgery.*[26, 27, 28] Preliminary clinical data suggest a method of action by which ibuprofen-type drugs may have a negative effect on joint and tissue health: they adversely affect the body's balance of prostaglandins, a family of fatty acids involved in the body's inflammation processes.[29]

Although NSAIDs reduce the signs and symptoms of osteoarthritis and rheumatoid arthritis and bring pain relief to millions of people suffering other inflammatory disorders, they "do not eliminate underlying disease. Disease-modifying antirheumatic drugs also bring relief, but these drugs are often ineffective and not well tolerated. Failure to provide long-term benefits combined with the high toxicity of most of the disease-modifying agents has prompted a search for more effective treatments."[30]

Drugs (including probably dexamethasone) used in the treatment of arthritis and other chronic pain conditions also have the potential of depleting the blood of another important nutrient, sulfate, which is necessary to the body's production of cartilage cells called glycosaminoglycans, and may be especially necessary in common arthritis-related pain.

Indeed, the body is already not producing enough sulfur-derived glycosaminoglycans when it is suffering from chronic pain conditions, especially arthritis, osteoarthritis, and other inflammatory conditions. Under the influence of these drugs, the body produces even fewer glycosaminoglycans. Those that are produced tend to be sulfate-depleted and inferior in quality. This results in further joint deterioration, and is intrinsically in opposition to healing.

Yet, because humans have naturally very low serum sulfate levels in their blood, they react extremely sensitively to sulfate depletion.

The very drugs intended to help damage the joint even more by depleting the body of sulfate.

Quite apart from the use of NSAIDs, cortisone-type medications, and other drugs–the usual treatments for pain are safe and helpful. The trouble is, they may not be able to make-up for the long-term tissue or joint deterioration that often accompanies chronic pain conditions. These safe and somewhat effective pain treatments include the use of moist heat or cold packs, exercise, stretching, and weight loss when necessary, as well as various capsaicin, salicylate and ibuprofen topical creams. We believe that these are excellent strategies, although most doctors tend not to place enough emphasis on diet and nutritional supplements, instead preferring the use of the types of drugs that we have discussed in this chapter.

It is with the choice of drugs over our proven natural agents for long-term use that we believe pain doctors are all too often going down a dead end street with dire consequences for patients.

No wonder J.M. Kremer, a rheumatologist from Albany Medical College, lamented in *Geriatrics*:

"Therapeutic advances have been made . . . but patients (and sometimes physicians) may become frustrated at the apparent lack of breakthrough treatments."[31]

There are dire consequences to a lifetime of painkillers. The damage may be as obvious as a hospital admission for bleeding of the gastrointestinal tract, ulcers, kidney or liver toxicity. But there is a more subtle damage, too. Even if not overtly obvious, weeks, if not months or years, spent on painkillers gnaw away at the spirit, at the mind of the user. Pain can be a chance to transcend, but with painkillers can also dampen life, create depression, and reliance on yet further drugs. The spiral can easily go out of control.

We should be thankful, indeed, for the opportunity to learn about the healing powers of systemic oral enzymes.

"No doubt, these fast acting drugs relieve pain. Believe it or not, unfortunately, that is not all that they do. They inhibit the repair processes your joints desperately require in order to effect their healing. On the other hand, our recommended natural healing agents relieve pain and stimulate cartilage regrowth, a potentially superior health strategy that all patients should know about. Indeed, what we advocate is not medicine as usual."

"*Therapeutic advances have been made in rheumatoid arthritis, but patients (and sometimes physicians) may become frustrated at the apparent lack of breakthrough treatments. Some rheumatoid arthritis drugs, such as methotrexate, hold the specter of increased cancer risk.***"**

Bottom Line

* NSAIDs and other painkillers offer quick pain relief, but they do not address the underlying condition and may even hasten the degeneration of tissues.
* Use NSAIDs and other painkillers, if necessary for quick pain relief under acute conditions. Try to avoid their use beyond two or three days.
* The long-term complications associated with NSAIDs and other painkillers can be extremely serious, including gastrointestinal bleeding, ulcers, kidney and liver toxicity, as well as addiction and psychological disturbances.
* For long-term pain, prefer systemic oral enzymes.

Part II

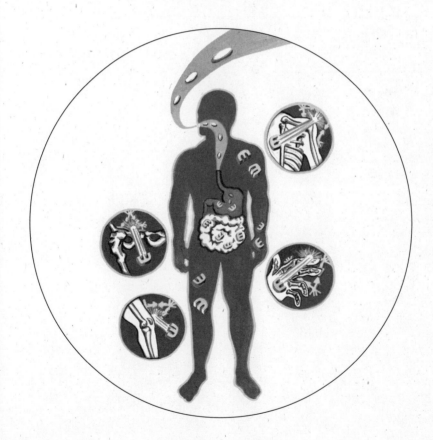

5

Systemic Oral Enzymes and Pain Relief

Michael is a 48-year-old baby boomer with baby boomer problems–a baby boomer wife, five post-boomer kids (all daughters), and plenty of financial uncertainty. Getting the daily tasks done is hard enough, but keeping the muscle and fat where it is suppose to be is an unrelenting task.

Michael has had two knee surgeries from basketball trauma about 10 years ago. In fact, the initial trauma involved a compression fracture that virtually destroyed the integrity of the medial compartment of the right knee. He put on about 12 pounds after surgery and hasn't been able to get it off. Previously, he relied on running to sort of fix his weight when it would start to go up. For a long, long time, Michael was depressed, stiff, and unable to run. There did not seem to be an easy answer.

Part of the answer came when Michael started taking glucosamine sulfate three times a day. There was less pain, less barometric pressure, and a better ability to move about. But running? This was not even a consideration.

Michael then started taking systemic oral enzymes on a regular basis–10 to 15 Wobenzym® N tablets daily in three divided doses. Sounds like a lot, doesn't it? This was the amount recommended to get started to be sure that any microtrauma did not result in having to stop the exercise program. The results? Michael is now running five miles daily on the treadmill (no elevation yet). His weight has dropped. The stiffness is minimal to none. The pain in his knee is gone. His appetite is good—but no longer excessive. His energy is high. "I know that the oral enzymes made a big difference," he says. "I can do things physically I thought I would never be able to do again. I feel great. I feel healthier than ever before."

What are enzymes anyway?

Already during the dim and distant past, enzymes were used by mankind. It was known that grape juice or the juices stemming from specific grains could be altered into a fluid whose consumption brought about pleasant sensations. This wondrous transformational process later came to be known as fermentation. And it was occurring throughout the biological world. Indeed, we would not have life today without this process. It took a long time, however, to discover the inner workings of this process.

Today, we have grounds for assuming that there are thousands of catalytic processes taking place between tissues and fluids in living plants and animals. These all result from the power of enzymes!

Today we know that an enzyme is any of various types of proteins which act as catalysts to speed up the body's biochemical processes. Without enzymes, life could not exist. Enzymes are the tools that create life. All living material contains enzymes. Enzymes control the chemical reactions of all organisms, big or small. Enzymes act as catalysts and they work in a "lock and key" manner to change the structure of molecules by splitting them or combining them.

More than three thousand different enzymes have now been identified in the human body and registered with the world's official enzyme commission. They build new proteins, cells, tissues, and organs, and also tear down these same tissues.

Enzymes are derived from several different sources. Enzymes such as bromelain and papain are derived from plants, particularly pineapples and papayas, respectively. Other enzymes, such as amylase and lipase, are derived from bacteria. The enzymes trypsin and pancreatin are derived from porcine pancreas.

We all need optimal enzyme activity throughout our lives if we are to enjoy fantastic health. Unfortunately, however, the moderate temperatures at which most foods are cooked destroy enzymes. Although enzymes are found most active in raw or lightly cooked foods, most people won't eat raw foods, especially meat which provides several important enzymes.

What's more, the majority of food people consume today is *both processed* and *cooked* at extremely high temperatures, reducing dietary enzyme levels even more. For these reasons, people receive very few enzymes from their diets, and, in effect, are suffering effects of low enzymes. Other medical experts point out that young people have much more enzyme activity than older people whose ability to manufacture enzymes diminishes with age. Perhaps this is the reason inflammatory diseases become so prevalent as people age.

Inflammation: At The Heart of Many Chronic Disease States

Systemic oral enzymes excel at quelling inflammation. This is important because inflammation is at the heart of many chronic disease states–including pain conditions as well as heart disease. Systemic oral enzymes support and accelerate the natural inflammatory process without letting it get out of control. Enzyme mixtures work by hindering or lessening excessive inflammatory reactions. They have been shown to help:

* Break down proteins in the blood that cause inflammation by facilitating their removal via the blood stream and lymphatic system.
* Remove "fibrin," the clotting material that prolongs inflammation.
* Clear up edema (excess water) in the areas of inflammation.
* Counteract chronic, recurrent inflammation, a primary cause of chronic degenerative joint and other diseases.

During disease states and during ordinary aging, the body produces damaged or pathologic proteins. These are sometimes called immune complexes. These circulating complexes of damaged proteins accumulate in body parts such as the blood vessels, joints, and other tissues where they become systemic irritants, causing inflammation, and delaying the healing process. Unfortunately, in chronic disease states, the cleaning capacity of the body is reduced, and bad proteins (the circulating immune complexes) can accumulate. In cases where there is acute inflammation, such as rheumatoid arthritis or sinusitis, these immune complexes have grown so much in number they have taken up permanent residence in the body's tissues.

Systemic oral enzymes destroy these bad proteins and immune complexes, helping the immune system to do its job better by removing inflammatory substances. Think of systemic oral enzymes as a co-worker and partner in a healthy immune system that, in turn, helps with chronic pain conditions.

That is because this pathological process, involving bad proteins and immune complexes, occurs in many different types of chronic pain conditions such as rheumatoid arthritis, lupus, diabetes mellitus, sinusitis, thrombophlebitis, prostatitis, and many other conditions–all related by the fact that they represent out-of-control inflammatory states. These are very common age-related diseases, and many people use enzymes as a lifetime helper to deal more effectively with these conditions.

How Systemic Oral Enzymes Relieve Inflammation

A quality systemic enzyme preparation is a biological response modifier that works with the body's own immune defense system to moderate the inflammatory process.

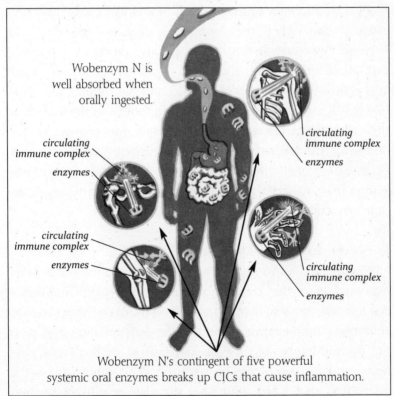

Wobenzym N is well absorbed when orally ingested.

circulating immune complex

enzymes

circulating immune complex

enzymes

circulating immune complex

enzymes

circulating immune complex

enzymes

Wobenzym N's contingent of five powerful systemic oral enzymes breaks up CICs that cause inflammation.

In many common auto-inflammatory conditions such as arthritis, the immune system becomes hyperstimulated and begins to malfunction.

Although medical science is unsure of the exact reason, scientists have observed that, for some reason, the body's immune system begins to form apparently unneeded antibodies. An antibody is any of numerous protein molecules produced as a primary immune defense by the immune system's lymphocytes; it is the B cells that produce antibodies that attack and defuse foreign substances in the body.

Each antibody has a uniquely shaped site that usually combines with a foreign substance such as a virus or toxin and disables it. But, when the immune system malfunctions and becomes hyperactivated, it overreacts and produces antibodies that attack even seemingly harmless substances in the blood. This causes the formation of irritating circulating immune complexes (CICs) that are so misshapen and foreign to the body that they themselves are attacked by the immune system. Nearby otherwise healthy tissues may also be impacted, causing further exacerbation of the immune firestorm. This causes an immune system that is attacking both its own cells and the tissues of the body, resulting in chronic inflammation.

Enzymes Accelerate Elimination of CICs

Rheumatoid arthritis is but one of many immune and inflammatory diseases that commonly cause chronic pain conditions—but few conventional treatments address the underlying systemic condition. Most treatments reduce the inflammation and pain but do nothing to start the healing process. In this sense, systemic oral enzymes may be superior. Their influence on the immune system is profound. They stimulate healthy production of messenger immune cells (cytokines) that quench inflammation and rev up immunity to produce a cleansing effect, helping to cleave or break up circulating immune complexes (CICs) at the center of the body's immune/inflammation firestorm. Eventually, the body's inflammation levels are markedly reduced, enabling the pain sufferer to once again resume normal activity.

Immunological Effects— Frequently a Long-Term Benefit

Beyond inflammation, systemic enzyme therapy also has a regulatory effect on various phases of the immunological system. The stimulation of macrophages and killer cells, as well beneficial effects on the regulation of cytokines and other messenger cells involved in immune function, are also some of the long-term benefits from systemic oral enzyme therapy.

The treatment of a disturbed immune system, however, often requires patience and time. The effects of systemic oral enzyme therapy on the immune system and treatment of autoimmune diseases involving rheumatoid factors are profound but may involve weeks or even months.

Summary of Effects of Systemic Oral Enzymes

❖ *Systemic oral enzymes have an anti-inflammatory effect*
They degrade cell fragments and mediators of inflammation and infection.
They degrade protein molecules which have been transported from the blood stream and have penetrated into the tissues to subsequently cause the development of edema and exacerbate inflammation.

❖ *Proteolytic enzymes improve the flow characteristics of the blood*
They increase the flexibility of red blood cells, improving their ability to pass through the arteries.
They inhibit the aggregation of platelets.
They increase the fibrinolytic activity in the blood to help prevent abnormal clotting.

❖ *Systemic oral enzymes support degradation of pathological immune complexes*
They stimulate the ability of the immune system to break-down pathogenic immune complexes that may also exacerbate inflammation.

❖ *Systemic oral enzymes have a regulatory effect on the immune system.*
They activate macrophages and natural killer cells. The result is that the body's immune system is better equipped in numbers to deal with inflammation by cleansing itself of cellular debris and to quickly neutralize errant cancer cells.
They regulate of the metabolism of cell mediator substances such as tumor necrosis factor and interleukins. These tough cops kill dangerous cells and tissues circulating in the body–including foreign proteins, and inflammatory debris.

❖ *Systemic oral enzymes increase the tissue permeability for antibiotics and possibly other drugs*
They synergize doctor–prescribed drugs, improving their clinical outcome

❖ *Systemic oral enzymes accelerate the healing process*
They support the cleansing of the tissues and promote better circulation.
They stimulate formation of new, healthy tissue.

But, Why Haven't I Heard About Systemic Oral Enzymes?

Obviously and sadly, your doctor may not know about systemic oral enzymes. It is not trendy to accept European studies as the basis for clinical opinion. Historically, the primary bias may lay with the Food and Drug Administration (FDA), or arguably with our medical education system which tends not to teach nutrition or use of vitamin and mineral therapies. Also of note, is that many of our most noteworthy American medical journals have until recently avoided articles on nutrition, feeling they more aptly should be published elsewhere or not at all. Then again, some doctors feel extremely uncomfortable recommending a food rather than drugs. What is important is that this is beginning to change. Not only are many of the drug and herbal companies located in Europe capable of exerting their financial clout with massive advertising campaigns in select American media outlets, they are all acting as global companies. They are advertising and selling by international routes, and beginning multinational clinical trials. By reading this book, you too are on the cutting edge of modern medicine and healing. What's more, our information systems are now global. You can now search the European data banks as well as Medline by simply getting on the Internet and surfing. The information is there and available and the quality of the data is as good, if not better, than much of the research done in America.

It is our opinion that systemic oral enzymes offer the first mainstream long-term treatment option with proven healing and safety. This is especially true when compared to corticosteroids and less potent anti-inflammatories. It is not our position or intent to disparage other claims, and we recognize the occasional specific need for these latter agents, but for mainstream prevention, and reversal, systemic oral enzymes make more sense and costs less cents. The toxicity of the NSAIDs and corticosteroids is well known particularly with regard to upset stomach (epigastritis), kidney disease (interstitial nephritis), and liver damage (hepatocellular mitochondrial damage). We present this information as a physician and consumer advocate, hoping that your healing path will be a quick journey without wasting precious time or valuable dollars on unproved therapies. We feel that this information is especially important because it comes at a time when pharmaceutical companies, according to *The Wall Street Journal*, are likely to be launching heavy advertising campaigns for prescription drugs on television and other forms of mass media.[32] You, the consumer, are likely to be asking your physician for these drugs because you saw them on TV, rather than ask for systemic oral enzymes because you have searched out the data. In a mass media campaign, it is unlikely the risks will receive equal time and print size with the benefits of these new drug therapies. It is imperative that consumers be informed. Health knowledge is more important today than ever. By being informed, you are actually helping doctors to do their job better.

We also know that many doctors will continue to remain skeptical that natural substances like systemic oral enzymes work as well as their medical drugs. They will continue to argue that systemic oral enzymes have no scientific evidence because they will not accept findings from the European clinical trials. It is very interesting that reliable knowledge stops just east of New York, according to the FDA.

What Do I Tell My Doctor if I Want to Start to Use System Oral Enzymes?

Systemic oral enzymes are completely safe. Because they are so safe and without virtually any drug interactions whatsoever, many people use systemic oral enzymes without medical advice from their doctor or other health professional. In many cases, this is acceptable. Other people, however, may find it more beneficial to work with their doctor or other health professional who can act as their "coach" and who can help them to design a specific, comprehensive healing program. What's more, your informed health care advisor can help you to measure your healing progress with objective benchmarks by measuring quantitatively improvements in mobility and freedom from pain.

Systemic oral enzymes have been proven to be extremely safe. Still, if you are on a medical drug or involved in any medical procedures or have any possible health concerns, it is always best to talk with a trusted, qualified health care professional. If you have a unique health situation, we urge you to be sure to work with a health professional when designing a supplement program. Having said this, some doctors may be open and some not to your using this perfectly safe healing agent.

If your doctor is reluctant to have you start using systemic oral enzymes, you may wish to locate a doctor who will be of more help to you. Consumers who find themselves without adequate professional advice in their community should be sure to go to your Resources section in the back of this book to find sources for doctors in their area who are familiar with the use of systemic oral enzymes.

Show your doctor this book, if needed. Throughout the course of this book, we have endeavored to present solid, factual information aimed at the mainstream medical community, particularly medical consumers and their care givers with the hope that doctors will be enlightened and give pause to reflect on whether it really should be "business as usual" when it comes to the treatment of their patients with pain and related inflammatory conditions.

Education is at the heart of what doctors are doing. If we have done this, we will have helped people, and that is what medicine, in its most noble form, is all about.

P.S. If, however, your health professional continues to ignore the evidence that I will shortly present, it is important to seek a health professional who will take an active interest in your healing work.

Now, let's look at how systemic oral enzymes can help with specific pain and other related conditions.

6

Systemic Oral Enzymes and Arthritis

Health is mobility. If you don't have mobility, you don't have health. It's really that simple. Imagine, if you will, that your joints are like a "rusty door hinge," creaking, sticking and just not moving. This is what happens with arthritis. Other people liken the pain of arthritis to a fire in the joints, burning, inflaming their tissues. Others use words like "gritty," "grinding" and "popping" to describe the condition of their inflamed joints.

Imagine if you would that your joints are like a "rusty hinge"– creaking, sticking–that just won't move. No matter how patients describe their own individual cases of arthritis, the fact is that this condition is painful and debilitating. It is a robber of joy and happiness, and one that is becoming increasingly prevalent among the American population, especially among the aging "baby boomer" generation. Rheumatoid arthritis, in fact, is commonly one of the most difficult diseases pain specialists see.

Imagine, if you will the following images either now in your life or perhaps when you are older and in your fifties, sixties, or beyond . . . Imagine . . .

- ❖ being at a party with a lively band, yet not being able to dance;
- ❖ sitting at home on a glorious fall evening but unable to take an evening walk;

❖ not being able to hike up to your favorite vista or mountain peak to see the clouds blowing in over the mountains,
or the ocean or prairie lands spread below;

❖ feeling the pounding pain from the concrete that you walk
on–as though your legs and feet are drumming;

❖ reaching for a package of scotch tape or another small
item, but being unable to actually grip or even open it
because your hands and fingers are so inflamed that they
have lost their flexibility and strength.

These images are real. This is what happens with arthritis.
These are images to which we can all relate. They affect everyday
people–possibly you or someone you know.

What's more, such problems, like those that we've described,
happen far more often than you might think. Finally, however,
thanks to systemic oral enzymes and other supporting nutrients
and health strategies, we may finally be able to do something so
that these limitations will not be as common in the future as they
are today and predicted to be.

Yes, health is mobility, and our loss of mobility affects mental, as well as physical, health.

Indeed, arthritis is a word we are all likely to get to know as
we get older. It has been estimated that as many as four of five
of the eighty million baby boomers in America today will eventually require help for one form or another of arthritis. Arthritis
is America's number one enemy when it comes to loss of mobility, one of the very attributes we often take for granted, and that
makes so much of life worth living. Fortunately, we can now do
something to protect our bodies from crippling arthritis. But wait
a minute. We're getting ahead of ourselves.

First things first . . .

What is Arthritis, anyway?

The nineteenth century London physicist Sir Archibald Gerrod described and named this widespread crippler that today we call arthritis.

Arthritis, literally translated, means "fire in the joints." In its simplest definition, arthritis is an inflammatory disease of the joints. Although more than one-hundred different forms of the disease have been identified in the field of rheumatology (the scientific name of the study of arthritis), two types are most prevalent: osteoarthritis and rheumatoid arthritis. Generally speaking, we can divide the types of arthritis into even two larger categories: inflammatory, immune-related arthritis and simple osteoarthritis. Also, even though arthritis comes in more than a hundred varieties, most forms of this disease include some joint

---

The Five Most Common Forms of Arthritis

Osteoarthritis: The most common form of arthritis, osteoarthritis affects from 15 to 20 million Americans–usually over age 45.

Rheumatoid arthritis: An inflammatory and immune-mediated disease, rheumatoid arthritis, also known simply as RA, affects up to about eight million people–usually women.

Gout: Usually associated with lifestyle and diet, gout affects some one million persons–usually men.

Ankylosing spondylitis (spinal arthritis): Causing immobility of the back, and often the shoulders and neck, ankylosing spondylitis, an inflammatory form of arthritis, affects more than 300,000 people–usually men. Again, systemic oral enzymes can help tremendously.

Systemic Lupus Erythematosus: Technically not an arthritis but an immune-related form of arthralgia often affecting the hip joints, systemic lupus erythematosus, also known as SLE, affects about 131,000 people–usually women. Systemic oral enzymes can be very helpful to patients with lupus.

degeneration and inflammation as part of their pathology. That is why a substance such as systemic oral enzymes is so important.

❝ Arthritis comes in more than a hundred varieties. Most forms of this disease include some joint degeneration and inflammation as part of their pathology. That is why a substance such as systemic oral enzymes is so important. ❞

Rheumatoid Arthritis

Rheumatoid arthritis is a chronic disease of the joints character-ized by alternating periods of active inflammation and absence of symptoms, both of variable duration.[33] Some of the symptoms include a sense of utter fatigue and weakness, running a very slight fever. The joints may become just a little stiff at first, but a few weeks later they become much stiffer and swollen. The stiff-ness and swelling may start in the small joints like the fingers and wrists but progress to larger joints and afflict both the joints and bodily organs. This is a total disease. It affects the body inside and outside. Interestingly, symmetrical joints such as the hands, wrists and ankles, are often hit first with an attack. The joints may even be "hot" to the touch. About one third of rheumatoid arthritis patients get luckier than most, and only a single joint area or two are affected, but for most, the pain will be spread throughout the entire body.

About eight million Americans have rheumatoid arthritis. The usual age at which it strikes is in the 20 to 40 age group.[34] In terms of gender differentiation, rheumatoid arthritis is most likely to strike women aged 36 to 50, according to the National Rheumatism Foundation. The next major target is men 45 to 60. Some children and teenagers suffer various forms of rheumatoid arthritis.

In rheumatoid arthritis, the immune system is out of control and turns on the body. Although medical science is unsure of the exact cause of rheumatoid arthritis, we do know that for some reason the body's immune system begins to form apparently unneeded antibodies that cause a chronic inflammation of the joints. An antibody is any of numerous protein molecules produced as a primary immune defense by the immune system's lymphocytes; it is the B cells that produce antibodies which attack and defuse foreign substances in the body; each antibody has a uniquely shaped site that combines with a foreign substance such as a virus or toxin and disables it. Eventually, however, these antibodies form large immune complexes that are so misshapen and foreign to the body itself that they themselves are attacked by the immune system or simply cannot be eliminated. Eventually, this causes an immune system that is attacking the body's own tissues, resulting in inflammation and joint destruction. Eventually, this congregation of aberrant immune cells in a specific area of the body, such as the joints, causes inflammation. In rheumatoid arthritis, the thin membrane surrounding the joints (synovium) becomes swollen and extremely inflamed. As these attacks continue to occur, the bones and joint tissues are weakened and eventually destroyed, destroying the integrity of the joint, including the cartilage which provides a cushioning effect. This battle within the immune system is likely to spread throughout the body, damaging and killing off the red blood cells. This then leads to the constellation of symptoms within the body, including weakness, fatigue, and swelling.

The formation of these new antibodies may be heightened due to a variety of influences on a person's health. Your genes, for example, may make you vulnerable to foreign toxins and pathogens such as food allergies and biological pathogens such as bacteria and viruses, which can initiate an immune firestorm. However, other influences under your direct control include your lifestyle and diet and these can potentiate the firestorm, as can allergies.

Small joints are usually most affected, including knuckles and toe joints. Yet, the wrists, knees, ankles, and the small interlocking joints of the neck can also be targeted. However, less known is that this inflammation can spread to the eyes, heart, lungs, and blood vessels.

Some experts believe that rheumatoid arthritis can be caused by allergens, especially those in the diet, combined with a permeable intestinal wall (leaky gut wall syndrome) that allows large undigested food particles to pass through and initiate the immune response that eventually leads to the disabling and painful inflammation associated with rheumatoid arthritis. James Braly, M.D., medical director of Immuno Labs, Inc., of Fort Lauderdale, Florida, notes:

"Five to ten years ago, it would have been heresy to state that allergens could induce arthritis and that, by the elimination of those allergens, the arthritis would go into remission. Now it's accepted among most rheumatologists and allergists that some people do have allergy-induced arthritis. A primary cause of most rheumatoid arthritis appears to be delayed food allergy and the often related problem of abnormal permeability of the intestinal wall [leaky gut syndrome]."[35]

According to this theory, partially digested food particles pass through the intestinal wall into the bloodstream. These unintentional "invaders" are then deposited in the body's joint and other tissues where they can cause an inflammatory response as the body's immune system mobilizes to disarm them.

It is not as well known, but bacterial infections may be at the root of some cases of rheumatoid arthritis. Other microbial invaders including protozoa, yeast, and fungus can also cause or aggravate arthritis. Finally, some medical drugs such as diuretics may trigger arthritis. And for some, albeit a small percentage, their condition may simply be genetic, that is inherited.

Rheumatoid arthritis has a very subtle method of attack. You might not even know for an extended period of time that your body is under attack. In its *Family Medical Guide*, the American Medical Association expertly describes the disease's onset:

"Rheumatoid arthritis may begin without obvious symptoms in the joints. Over several weeks or even months you
may feel generally ill, listless, and without appetite. You are
likely to lose weight and to have vague muscular pains and
possibly a low-grade fever. Only later do you develop the
joint symptoms that are typically characteristic of rheumatoid arthritis. In other cases, the inflammation flares up sud-
denly, without previous symptoms of any kind. When your
joints are affected, they become red, warm, swollen, tender
to the touch, painful to move, and stiff. The stiffness is usually most noticeable first thing in the morning. As you move
and exercise the joints, the pain and stiffness gradually
become less severe." [36]

Although rheumatoid arthritis is a complex disease whose causes are not extremely well understood, help is available.

One of the most important applications today for systemic oral enzymes is with arthritis, particularly the most difficult-to-treat joint disease such as rheumatoid arthritis.

Of particular note to parents is their ability to help has been shown to extend to children's juvenile chronic arthritis. In fact, we have also seen altogether too many patients, both adults and chil-dren, who have come to systemic oral enzymes as a last resort because they have not received the kind of help their bodies crave.

The drugs that doctors commonly prescribe such as non-steroidal anti–inflammatory drugs (NSAIDs), corticosteroids, gold salts and methotrexate are extremely toxic and can result in damage to the bones and joint matrix. And when it comes to young children and inflammatory diseases, we still have only these extremely toxic drugs. It is tough to see young children on corticosteroids, but doctors try to control the complications the best that they can. We urge you to try systemic oral enzymes. As you read through this chapter, you will be filled with true hope and excitement over the prospect of finally stepping off the drug treadmill.

Osteoarthritis

Another name for osteoarthritis, *arthrosis*, literally means "degenerative joint disease." This certainly characterizes osteoarthritis which usually becomes more apparent in older people, especially in the larger, weight–bearing joints, including the hips, knees, and spine.

Under the age of 45, osteoarthritis is more common in men. However, after age 45 it is ten times more common in women than men.[37] Forty million Americans have some form of osteoarthritis from mild to severe, including 80 percent of people over age 50. Some 20 million Americans suffer from disabling osteoarthritis. This number is likely to increase by three or four times over the next several decades. Also, people in specific types of occupations may be more affected than others. "Many ballet dancers get it in their feet after years of standing on their toes. Football players have also been particularly susceptible to problems with their joints as a result of repeated trauma and injuries to the joints that occur during games."[38]

Stages of the Osteoarthritis Process

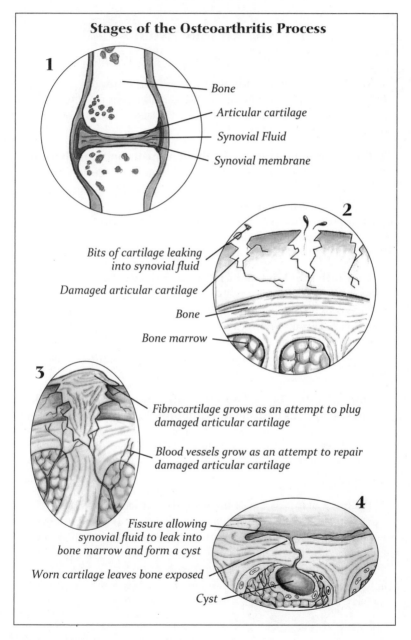

1
— Bone
— Articular cartilage
— Synovial Fluid
— Synovial membrane

2
Bits of cartilage leaking into synovial fluid
Damaged articular cartilage
Bone
Bone marrow

3
Fibrocartilage grows as an attempt to plug damaged articular cartilage
Blood vessels grow as an attempt to repair damaged articular cartilage

4
Fissure allowing synovial fluid to leak into bone marrow and form a cyst
Worn cartilage leaves bone exposed
Cyst

Five Arthritis Myths

Take this quiz and test your arthritis acumen.

1. You'll get osteoarthritis if you live long enough.

False. Osteoarthritis is *not* inevitable. You can alter your diet, exercise, and use nutritional supplements that will dramatically reduce your risk of ever suffering a debilitating joint disease.

2. There's nothing you can do about arthritis once you have it.

False. Systemic oral enzymes, combined with other ingredients, provide a safe, natural and proven method for relieving pain and rebuilding cartilage. What's more, additional changes in diet and lifestyle, together with intelligent use of nutritional supplements, can provide help to a great many arthritis sufferers whether they are suffering from osteoarthritis or rheumatoid arthritis or other forms of the disease.

3. Pain killers relieve pain without side effects.

False. Evidence suggests that pain killers may be used in higher and higher doses over time and cause long-term damage to the cartilage and bones by altering the body's cartilage cells' metabolism. What's more, most OTC pain killers pose chronic toxicity problems to the kidneys and liver, and they virtually all cause micro-bleeding in the gastrointestinal tract.

4. Only people who've had traumatic injuries or who work in professions like professional football get osteoarthritis.

Not true! A concert pianist, who spends his days hunched over his keyboard, may also suffer from arthritis. Ballet dancers are also known to suffer higher than normal rates of osteoarthritis. Anyone can get osteoarthritis.

5. If I have arthritis I will have to give up an active life.

Not so. In fact, most people with arthritis can go on to live relatively, if not fully, active lives. Exercise, when done intelligently, is a healing elixir for your joints. Exercise forces fluids to be exchanged, moving nutrients in, debris and toxins out. Furthermore, modern medical technologies, if absolutely necessary, such as hip or knee replacement can return lost mobility to arthritis sufferers.

In osteoarthritis, the smooth lining of a joint, known as the articular cartilage, begins to flake and crack. With the loss of this protective cartilage, the underlying bone becomes thickened and distorted. Eventually, this may lead to episodes of pain, swelling, and stiffness in the affected joint. These episodes may be chronic or occur at intervals of months or years. Some people may not even notice the swelling. While in other cases, affected joints may become extremely knobby and enlarged. Sometimes the pain seems to move from the affected joint to other areas of the body. This is known as referred pain. As one team of experts notes, "Osteoarthritis of the hip is sometimes felt most painfully in the front of the thigh and knee."[39]

What are the symptoms of osteoarthritis? Morning stiffness is one of the first. Pain after prolonged use of a certain joint is an early sign. The pain becomes worse with prolonged activity, better with rest. Loss of range of motion is another. The disturbing sense that your joints have crackled is a symptom that indicates the disease is worsening (crepitus). This is most likely to occur in the hips or knees. However, as the condition progresses, people may experience more pain–even without motion.

Many doctors say osteoarthritis is inevitable given the daily wear and tear on the body's joints. This just isn't true. We can make conditions much tougher for our joints by our own personal lifestyle habits. Due to our increasingly inactive lifestyles and fatty diets, our joints are being asked to carry far more weight than ever before. Too many of us are junk food and television addicts. The joints just can't hold up to obesity and eventually do wear out. *One-third of us are obese.* Exercise and diet are key, as is regular use of quality healing supplements. Again, systemic oral enzymes are critical for enhancing the body's healing response.

The Miracle of Systemic Oral Enzymes

Now, thanks to a mountain of evidence as high as Mt. Everest, we know that systemic oral enzymes may be one of the best medicines for both adults and children with difficult-to-treat inflammatory/joint conditions.

Enzymes Accelerate Elimination of CICs

Although rheumatoid arthritis is truly an immune and inflammatory disease, few conventional treatments address the underlying systemic condition. Most treatments reduce the inflammation and pain but do nothing to start the healing process. In this sense, enzymes may be superior. Their influence on the immune system is profound and stimulates once again healthy production of messenger immune

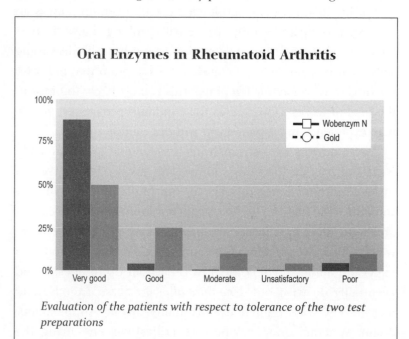

Evaluation of the patients with respect to tolerance of the two test preparations

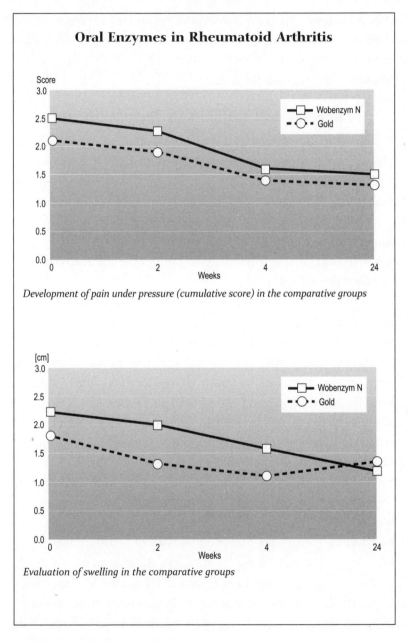

Development of pain under pressure (cumulative score) in the comparative groups

Evaluation of swelling in the comparative groups

cells (cytokines) that quench inflammation and rev up immunity to produce a cleansing effect, helping to cleave or break up circulating immune complexes (CICs) at the center of the body's RA immune/inflammation firestorm.

Enzymes and Difficult-to-Treat Arthritis

Excellent early results using the patented enzyme formula Wobenzym" N were noted by researchers writing in 1985 in *Zeitschr. f. Rheumatologie*. In this study, patients took eight Wobenzym N tablets four times daily. Sixty-two percent of patients improved.[40]

A 1988 report in *Natur- und Ganzheitsmedizin* showed that the same formula can prevent further flare-ups and helps to lower levels of inflammatory-related circulating immune complexes in rheumatoid arthritis patients.[41]

Another study also published in *Natur- und Ganzheitsmedizin* in 1988 noted that Wobenzym N has demonstrated similar benefits to gold therapy but without toxic side effects.[42]

Wobenzym N will also be helpful with non-inflammatory active osteoarthritis, as has been shown for more than 20 years now. In one study among eighty patients Wobenzym N was pitted against the NSAID diclofenac.[43] Patients received either seven coated Wobenzym N tablets four times daily and two capsules or placebo or seven coated tablets of placebo four times daily and two 50 mg capsules of diclofenac. The groups were similar with respect to symptoms. An evaluation of all principal criteria examined revealed equivalent therapeutic results in both groups after four weeks. This means that even in cases of active osteoarthritis, Wobenzym N can be considered equivalent treatment.

Most recently, researchers from the Ukrainian Rheumatology Centre, in Kiev, tested Wobenzym on 78 patients with severe, crippling RA and who were using other prime treatment drugs.[41] Half

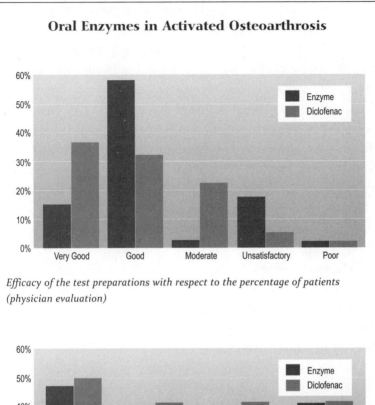

Efficacy of the test preparations with respect to the percentage of patients (physician evaluation)

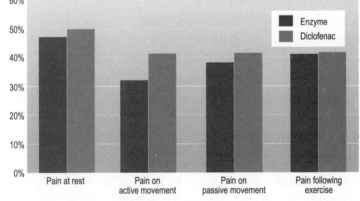

Improvement in symptoms in the comparative groups after four weeks of therapy

the patients had chronic fevers, some 23 percent had rheumatic nodules, and more than half were suffering from low hemoglobin/red blood cell counts. Many of these people had tried gold salts, methotrexate, and other non–steroidal anti–inflammatory drugs but to no avail, and some were even using canes and wheelchairs.

All of the RA patients showed a decrease in CIC concentrations, averaging between 28 and 42 percent, and decreases in rheumatoid factors. Twenty percent of patients reduced their NSAID doses by 50 to 75 percent. One patient stopped taking methotrexate and experienced a clinical remission of the disease. Morning stiffness scores improved. More than half the patients rated their treatment with Wobenzym as good, compared to only about a third of the patients using only medical drugs.

"The study results therefore confirm that Wobenzym is a new and quite effective antirheumatic agent, which also presents the properties of a second–line agent," said the Russian researchers at the Second Russian Symposium on Oral Enzyme Therapy in St. Petersburg, Russia, 1996.

At this same conference, researchers presented findings on Wobenzym N and juvenile arthritis. In the study, among 10 children from the Pediatric Clinic of the Institute of Rheumatology of the Russian Academy of Medical Science, 10 children with JCA were given five tablets three times a day.[45] They could also receive treatment with one NSAID in addition to Wobenzym. In the children, the number of actively inflamed joints was reduced from 44 to 15, especially in the second month. One youthful patient with psoriatic arthritis experienced a significant reduction in dermal signs of the disease. The drug proved effective generally after four to five months of treatment.

Additional Help for Arthritis

Systemic oral combination enzymes have a profound effect on immune- and inflammation–mediated diseases, particularly rheumatoid arthritis and lupus. Meanwhile, glucosamine can help to rebuild joint cartilage. Other nutrients such as calcium, Vitamin D_3, and turmeric can also help to stabilize the joint matrix and relieve inflammation. Let's look a little more closely at each integral component of this medically and scientifically supported system.

Glucosamine

A natural substance found abundantly in the human body, glucosamine is made from the combination of a sugar and an amine, a derivative of ammonia containing nitrogen and hydrogen atoms, explains Ray Sahelian, M.D., author of *Glucosamine and Chondroitin* (Avery 1998).

"Glucosamine is found largely in cartilage and plays an important role in its health and resiliency," he adds. "As we age, we lose some of the glucosamine and other substances in cartilage. This can lead to the thinning of cartilage and the onset and progression of arthritis."

A new Canadian study shows that glucosamine hydrochloride may have positive benefits. The results of the first North American study with glucosamine hydrochloride were presented at the July 1998 meeting of the 12th Pan–American Congress of Rheumatology in Montreal, Canada. Dr. Joseph Houpt, from Mount Sinai Hospital, University of Toronto, Canada, in cooperation with Dr. Allan Russell, from Brampton Pain Clinic in Brampton, Ontario, Canada, gave 47 individuals with osteoarthritis glucosamine hydrochloride 500 mg three times a day for eight weeks. They compared the results to a placebo group of 47 individuals. At the conclusion of the study, 49 percent of those receiving glucosamine noted benefits. "However," adds Dr. Sahelian, "it appears that there is a high placebo effect in osteoarthritis since 45 percent of those on placebo also reported feeling better. Part of the reason of the high response from the placebo group may be due to pre-study media hype. Patient expectations may have had a significant effect on the clinical responses."

The researchers noted an improvement in the knee examination of patients in the glucosamine group from the fourth to the eighth week. Dr. Russell adds, "The most impressive finding was the significant decrease in pain which started at the fourth week and accelerated with time. We closely examined the results of an arthritis symptom questionnaire and found the glucosamine group had a better response than the placebo group in 23 out of the 24 questions." Mild gastrointestinal side effects were seen in 12 percent in both groups.

Chondroitin Sulfate

Made up of chains of sugars with negative electrical polarities, chondroitin sulfates are found in cartilage where they create tiny reservoirs to attract and hold water in the proteoglycan mortar. They help to bring water, shape, and cushioning to cartilage.

Chondroitin sulfates inhibit destructive enzymes that breakdown cartilage and prevent the carrying of nutrients into the cartilage; they stimulate synthesis of proteoglycans, glycosaminoglycans, and collagen, which make-up healthy cartilage. They are manufactured from healthy cartilage.

Chondroitin sulfate is an extremely large molecule and not well absorbed in the body when taken orally.[46] What's more, glucosamine sulfate is far more massively proven as a healing agent in cases of arthritis. Nevertheless, there is a limited body of evidence supporting chondroitin sulfate's benefits in the arthritic healing process.

❖ In 1986, a French study, using oral chondroitin sulfates, found that it helped in the healing of arthritic cartilage better than pain medication.[47]

❖ A 1992 study focusing on oral chondroitin sulfates found improvement.[48]

❖ A 1996 study from the *Journal of Rheumatology* assessed the clinical efficacy of chondroitin sulfate in comparison with diclofenac. Patients treated with the NSAID showed prompt and plain reduction of clinical symptoms, which, however, reappeared after the end of treatment; in the chondroitin group, the therapeutic response appeared later in time but lasted for up to three months after the end of treatment.[49]

Most recently, W.B. Saunders published *Osteoarthritis and Cartilage* which presents new preliminary findings in non–peer reviewed abstract form on chondroitin sulfate and arthritis.

❖ In one recently published study, doctors from Hungary's National Institute of Rheumatology and Semmelweis Medical School looked at chondroitin sulfates among patients suffering osteoarthritis of the knee.[50] All were given either 800 mg of oral chondroitin sulfates or placebo and could also take pain killers such as paracetamol. Six months later, the chondroitin sulfate group experienced significant improvement and required less pain medicine.

❖ European researchers compared chondroitin sulfate with placebo in a three–month, double–blind multi–center study of 127 patients suffering osteoarthritis of the knees.[51] Patients taking 1,200 mg of the chondroitin sulfates either all at once or three times daily in divided doses enjoyed significant pain relief and improved mobility compared with the placebo group.

❖ In a year–long double-blind, placebo-controlled study, patients were given chondroitin sulfate or placebo.[52] The patients receiving chondroitin experienced significantly improved mobility and less swelling, instability and effusions. Six of the patients using chondroitin showed significantly smoother, thicker cartilage, a sign of improved health. The chondroitin group used less pain killer medication. "Chondroitin is a symptomatic slow acting drug for the treatment of knee osteoarthritis with a good clinical outcome," concluded the researchers.

❖ American and French researchers used X-ray analysis to determine whether chondroitin sulfate could halt progression of osteoarthritis joint degradation.[53] In this study, 42 men and women, ranging in age from thirty-five to seventy-eight, were given either 800 mg of oral chondroitin sulfate or placebo. After a year of supplementation, thickness of the femoro-tibial joint of the knee decreased significantly among patients using placebo, but not among patients taking chondroitin sulfate.

Vitamin D₃

Scientists continue to discover new functions of vitamin D. Among these new functions are those noted in the immune system. Experiments have illustrated that the autoimmune diseases of multiple sclerosis and rheumatoid arthritis can be successfully treated with the vitamin D hormone and its analogs.[54]

In several studies on patients with rheumatoid arthritis, an association of bone loss with a persistently high disease activity has been found. Researchers associated with the Department of Internal Medicine IV, Friedrich Schiller University of Jena, Germany, investigated the relation between disease activity and serum levels of vitamin D metabolites, parathyroid hormone (PTH), and parameters of bone turnover in patients with rheumatoid arthritis.[55] A total of 96 patients (83 women and 13 men) were divided into three groups according to disease activity measured by serum levels of C-reactive protein (CRP). The results indicate that high disease activity in patients with rheumatoid arthritis is associated with an alteration in vitamin D metabolism and increased bone loss. The decrease of vitamin D metabolites in these patients may contribute to a negative calcium balance and inhibition of bone formation. Furthermore, low levels of vitamin D metabolites suppressed activated T cells and accelerated the arthritic process in rheumatoid arthritis.

In a study reported in the *British Journal of Rheumatology*, twenty-five consecutive in-patients who had suffered from rheumatoid arthritis for at least five years were found to have a dietary intake of vitamin D universally well below recommended levels.[56] Pathological fractures, often initially unrecognized, had occurred in the lower limb bones of seven patients in the previous five years. Those with fractures of the leg bones had evidence of more pronounced osteoporosis and five of the seven had been taking oral corticosteroids. Those with the severest osteoporosis had lower serum levels of vitamin D metabolites than the rest.

Calcium

Supplemental calcium is crucial for healthy joint tissues, especially in cases of arthritis. Total serum calcium levels were investigated in a study of 394 patients with rheumatoid arthritis, 4490 healthy subjects, and 2609 inpatients at a district general hospital.[57] Patients with rheumatoid arthritis had lower mean calcium levels than healthy subjects, but had similar levels to inpatients at the district general hospital. Thirty-eight inpatients with rheumatoid arthritis at a hospital for rheumatic diseases had lower total calcium levels than all other groups.

To determine the adequacy of calcium, folic acid, vitamin E, zinc, and selenium intake in patients with rheumatoid arthritis, researchers associated with the Department of Rheumatology, Waikato Hospital, Hamilton, New Zealand, conducted an observational study on 48 patients (13 men, 35 women; mean age, 64.5 years) with RA attending a specialty clinic in New Zealand comparing their dietary intake as measured by a 5-day dietary survey with recommended dietary intake (RDI) guidelines.[58] Information on disease activity, functional ability, and drug therapy also was obtained. The percentage of patients who achieved the RDI was 23% for calcium, 46% for folic acid, 29% for vitamin E, 10% for zinc, and only 6% for selenium. Patients on methotrexate had a significantly reduced intake of folic acid as a percentage of RDI compared with those on other therapies. In contrast, dietary intake of iron and protein was largely adequate and unrelated to anemia. Patients with RA should receive dietary education or supplementation to bring up their intake of calcium, folic acid, vitamin E, zinc, and selenium, noted the researchers.

Willow

The history of aspirin can be traced back to ancient Egypt where extract of willow bark was used to treat inflammation, report researchers associated with the Unit of Chemoprevention, International Agency for Research on Cancer, Lyon, France.[59] The active component of the extract was identified as the glucoside of salicylic alcohol. Today, one of the most popular German phyto preparations for rheumatoid arthritis uses natural salicylates for their pain-relieving and anti-inflammatory effects.

Systemic Oral Enzymes Benefit Persons with Systemic Lupus Erythematosus (SLE or Lupus)

Systemic Lupus Erythematosus (SLE or lupus) most often strikes young women between the ages of 20 to 40. Technically not an arthritis but an immune–related form of arthralgia often affecting the hip joints, systemic lupus erythematosus, also known as SLE, affects about 131,000 people–usually women.

The condition is characterized by severe fatigue and a butterfly rash across the face; debilitating pain and swelling often occur in the hands, wrists, elbows, knees, ankles, or feet. There may also be morning stiffness in the joints. Other signs and symptoms of lupus include a worsening of the butterfly rash across the face following sun exposure; a pale or blue tinge to the fingers when exposed to cold; and possibly hair loss.

Lupus is a serious condition because it may also cause diseases of the internal organs, including the heart, brain, lungs, and kidneys, as well as bleeding, anemia, and chronic infections. With proper treatment, however, lupus can be controlled, and sufferers can expect normal life expectancy.

Diagnosing lupus is not always easy. While some 95 percent of patients with lupus will have a positive test for antinuclear antibody (+ANA), which is an abnormal blood protein, this test is not all that specific and approximately five to ten percent of older patients will have this antibody in the absence of lupus. What is needed to confirm the diagnosis is a finding of the "rimmed pattern" of the ANA, and a positive anti–double stranded DNA test. Sometimes, if renal disease is present, a kidney biopsy is required. Once the diagnosis is made, treatment is available. While lupus is usually not a primary cartilage destroying disease, patients with lupus become deconditioned and are put on high dose steroids for long periods of time, and their joints wear out sooner. Hence, nutri-

tional supplements, antioxidant therapy and specific joint sparing
activities must be part of the healing program.

A number of authors have suggested Wobenzym N could
prove highly effective in combination therapy for SLE.[60] Enzymes
help to dissolve circulating immune complexes and antibodies
that cause the severe inflammation of SLE. According to D.A.
Lopez, M.D., associate clinical professor of medicine at the
University of California at San Diego Medical School and co-
author of *Enzymes: The Fountain of Life*, animals suffering from
this inflammatory condition, when given combination enzymes,
have shown significant improvement.

We also have clinical evidence. In one study of SLE patients presented at the 1996 Russian Symposium, clinical and laboratory
immuno-inflammatory activity was found to decrease more quickly with Wobenzym N than with medical drugs, and in a number of
cases it was possible to reduce the dose or to improve the safety
and side effects profile of non-steroidal anti-inflammatory drugs
(NSAIDs), corticosteroids and second-line agents being used.[61]

In the study, 18 patients were selected. They were young people,
with an age range of 18 to 46; yet, already their lives were crippled
with kidney disease and severe inflammation.

In SLE patients given Wobenzym N, inflammatory activity of the
disease regressed more quickly during treatment than in patients not
treated with this natural medicine. This was shown by a decrease in
tendency to hemorrhage. There were decreases in CICs and ANAs.

Five patients taking Wobenzym N were able to reduce their
dose of Voltaren or prednisolone. This is important because these
drugs often pose serious complications.

Enzymes may be particularly important for SLE sufferers for
another reason: they've been strongly shown to help prevent
kidney disease and failure, both of which are commonly associ-

ated with SLE, according to August Heidland, M.D., and co-investigators reporting in a 1997 issue of *Kidney International.*[62]

In the January–March 2007 issue of the internationally respected *Like Sprava* journal, a research report noted the antioxidant effect of Wobenzym N applied to patients with kidney disease. "There is formation of free radicals in mesangial cells in patients with chronic glomerulonephritis, which increases destruction of renal tissue and enable autoimmune inflammation," the article stated. "The unbalance between activity of oxidizing and antioxidizing starts developing. It accelerates the progression of the disease." The article presented the author's assessment of the influence of the enzyme medication on the main indices of oxidizing and antioxidizing systems. "It was established the presence of antioxidant effect in Wobenzym medication. The use of this medication in combination with other drugs and without them enables restoration of the disturbed balance."

And in the October–December 2002 issue of the Russian language journal *Patologicheskaia fiziologiia i èksperimental'naia terapiia*, the English-language abstract reports that, "Patients with chronic glomerulonephritis (CG) develop disturbances of lipid blood spectrum leading to additional damage to renal structure. The existent methods of pathogenetic therapy have no effect on lipid imbalance. Recently, many autoimmune diseases have been treated with systemic enzyme therapy (SET). The authors studied SET effect in disturbed lipid metabolism in experimental glomerulonephritis. Experimental animals showed morphological and biochemical changes similar to those in CG of man. SET reduced renal tissue damage and symptoms of dyslipoproteinemia."

Again, a good choice for helping to maintain kidney, as well as overall, health.

Ankylosing Spondylitis

Ankylosing spondylitis is a severe, inflammatory arthritis of unknown cause. Its association with the gene linkage called HLA B27 strongly indicates that genetic factors are important in the expression of the disease. Evidence suggests that disease occurs when a genetically predisposed person comes into contact with certain bacteria (Klebsiella being a candidate), viruses, and environmental factors, not yet identified.

What is known is that you don't want to have this form of arthritis. It will make your life miserable giving you severe back pain, often moving into the middle and upper back area all the way up to the neck, sometimes to the point where movement in any direction is severely limited; for the sufferer, even turning his head, bending, or stooping may be difficult, if not nearly impossible, to do without great pain. For the sufferer, it is as if his spinal column is fused into place. Early morning stiffness and many other physical limitations accompany this condition. In its advanced form, you can get almost total immobilization of the spine resulting in what's called the straight "poker spine."

The joints of the spine, both discs and facet joints, get inflamed and can fuse. Why the spine reacts with osteophytic spurring, and fusion is unknown, but likely part of the healing response attempt to heal something or at least wall it off. Yet, it can't seem to arrest it.

At first, the sufferer may feel that he simply has a strained back. However, instead of getting better, his condition worsens. Mornings when the sufferer arises from bed can be particularly troubling with spinal pain that lasts for hours. Over time, the pain becomes greater, mobility is more limited, and the suffering can be extremely painful.

This very troubling condition affects some 300,000 people and is especially common in men. Activity and pain relievers are probably the best antidote to this painful, all too often debilitating condition. If the condition becomes severe, the sufferer's posture may become deformed.

Medical science is not sure about the causes of ankylosing spondylitis. One plausible theory attributes its onset to a tissue condition. People with it have tissues known as HLA–B27 that closely mimic in appearance a bacteria called Klebsiella which usually resides in the bowel and feeds on starchy carbohydrates and multiplies. The body produces antibodies that destroy healthy tissues that look like this bacteria including HLA–B27 cells. The end result is the deposition of fibrous tissues. This leads to stiff, painful, immobile joints and spine.[63]

However, about half of the people with this form of inflammatory arthritis also suffer arthritis of the hips and shoulders. Also, in some cases, the disease actually may "burn out" after a few years, disappearing as mysteriously as it first appeared.

While ankylosing spondylitis is most likely immunologically mediated and genetically driven, this doesn't mean that you have to let it ravage your joints. Stopping the inflammation and immunodysregulation may require corticosteroids and potent immunological drugs to get on top of the destruction, but rebuilding and preventing further downward spiraling is likely to involve antioxidant therapy and nutritional supplementation with systemic oral enzymes.

Reports have been made concerning the positive influence of oral enzymes on ankylosing spondylitis. In 1980, Reinbold reported of his astonishing therapeutic success in the treatment of a 35–year–old patient with the condition whose complete remission had persisted for at least 12 years.

This report and other case histories which have also pro-
gressed similarly led Dr. K.M. Goebel to test the effect of the
enzyme formula Mulsal®, an oral enzyme formula manufactured
by Mucos Pharma GmbH, also the manufacturer of Wobenzym
N, and very similar in composition to Wobenzym N. In this
study, the oral enzyme preparation was compared with
indomethacin in a randomized, clinical, double-blind study on
40 patients with this painful condition.[64] The cumulative pain
scores were evaluated statistically at the end of therapy. The
analgesic potency of the enzymes was found to be less than that
of the NSAID at the beginning of therapy–but was found to be
significantly superior after three months of therapy. The tolerance of the enzyme preparation was rated by physicians and
patients as "good," whereas tolerance was found to be "moderate"
for the NSAID.

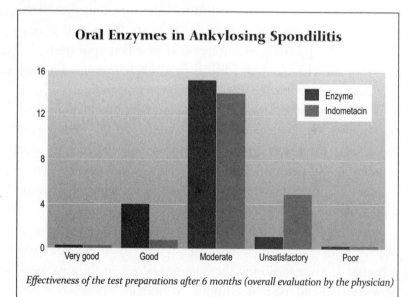

Oral Enzymes in Ankylosing Spondilitis

Effectiveness of the test preparations after 6 months (overall evaluation by the physician)

Bottom Line

Systemic oral enzymes can help:

* Slacken the development of arthritis
* Prevent deformations and invalidity
* Lessen pain
* Reduce inflammation
* Eliminate risk and worsening factors
* Preserve and improve the quality of life

Based on a thorough review of the pertinent literature, international experts have come up with the following guidelines to explain their benefits to you and your doctor.

* Systemic oral enzymes are a medication for the basic treatment in arthritis, acting on symptoms and having disease modifying properties.
* The symptomatic efficacy of systemic oral enzymes is comparable to NSAIDs.
* Systemic oral enzymes have no side effects (in contrast to NSAIDs).
* The onset of the symptomatic effect of arthritis may be delayed; however, after discontinuation of the treatment the beneficial effect continues for several weeks (in contrast to NSAIDs).
* All joints can be treated with systemic oral enzymes. The clinical efficacy of systemic oral enzymes has been demonstrated in different locations of the body: hip, knee, finger, spine.
* Virtually all common stages and types of arthritis can be treated, even very late ones. Ideally, early arthritis should be treated to stabilize cartilage metabolism and to normalize joint function.
* Patients of all ages can be treated.

❖ Systemic oral enzymes have a preventive and a therapeutic effect on osteoarthritis and also on traumatic events.

❖ The time for surgery can be temporarily postponed in case surgery is necessary. After surgical intervention, systemic oral enzyme treatment supports the regeneration of the joint tissues and also the contralateral joints which are overused due to the operated joints.

❖ Systemic oral enzymes improve quality of life in patients with all forms of arthritis.

How to Use . . .

For chronic pain relief, take three to five tablets three times daily 30 minutes before meals or not less than one hour after eating. For severe chronic pain, take five to ten tablets three times daily 30 minutes before meals or not less than one hour after eating.

During active flare-ups, increase dosage to five to ten tablets three to five times daily. Work with a health professional.

7
Systemic Oral Enzymes and Surgery

Another important area of application for systemic oral enzymes is for persons who must undergo various types of surgery. Indeed, if you're undergoing surgery, we would strongly urge you to consider using systemic oral enzymes before and after in order help stave off edema, inflammation, and excessive scarring and sclerosing of tissues, both internal and external. The clinical evidence that supports the use of systemic oral enzymes—Wobenzym N, in particular—is massive.

Doctors know that following trauma to the body, edema, hematomas (blood clots caused by tissue breakage), and preexisting inflammatory reactions make surgical intervention very difficult and can increase the risk of wound-healing impairment.

Meanwhile, postoperative swelling hampers blood flow and nutrients supplied to the tissues, thus increasing the likelihood of wound infections and delaying regeneration. The risk of embolisms and clotting complications also rises, due to the impaired microcirculation and additional immobility caused by injuries leading up to surgery and surgery itself.

Of course, very strong painkillers are sometimes required in acute situations, but the use of systemic oral enzymes can actually reduce your need for such medication, in some cases eliminating the need for stronger painkillers altogether.

Wobenzym N fulfills the highest standards and requirements for a substance that can safely and effectively modulate edema, inflammation and fibrinolytic action. Wobenzym N supports healthy blood viscosity and thereby improves microcirculation, and in this way supports the healing process. Since the formula also has an effect on the absorption of hematomas and an analgesic effect with hardly any undesirable side effects, Wobenzym N provides a comprehensive therapeutic approach.[65, 66, 67]

Because of these potent properties, systemic oral enzyme therapy therefore finds a broad range of application as a powerful health support agent in surgery, traumatology, and sports medicine. Wobenzym N has been used successfully for over 20 years in surgery and traumatology, and been described in numerous published reports and case histories. To a great extent, the advances in research on the inflammatory mechanisms and immunological reactions associated with use of Wobenzym N have yielded explanations for the clinically verified effects of enzyme therapy. Adding greatly to their validity, the success of oral enzymes in these fields of application has also been documented extensively in controlled clinical studies–the gold standard for all medicines.

Let's look at few of the most common uses of Wobenzym N for surgery.

Operative Dentistry

The prevention and treatment of edema and inflammation is of great importance in operative dental procedures. Due to the plentiful blood supply to the region of the mouth, the incidence of postoperative edema in surgical dental interventions is high. Numerous reports of the successful application of enzyme preparations in dentistry have been published.[68]

Dr. K. Vinzenz reported on the therapeutic usefulness of Wobenzym N in a randomized, placebo–controlled, double–blind study in *Die Quintessenz* in 1991.[69] Prior to surgical dental intervention, he prescribed ten coated tablets of Wobenzym N twice daily for 36 patients. In a similar regimen, 44 patients in the control group received placebo. This dosage was continued until the seventh postoperative day. None of the test subjects had received any preoperative therapy with other anti–inflammatory drugs.

Control examinations were performed two days preoperative, immediately prior to the operation, as well as on the first, third, fifth and seventh postoperative days. To make a clinical evaluation, Dr. Vinzenz determined the distance between the edge of the incisors with open mouth, the deviation of the midline with maximally opened mouth, as well as the thickness of the mucosal flap in the area of the periodontal membrane (i.e., the collagenous fibrous connective tissue between the cementum of the tooth and the socket in the jawbone in which the root or roots of the teeth are set). In addition to local inspection, Dr. Vinzenz analyzed the patients' blood serum in order to monitor the inflammatory process.

The laboratory data specific for inflammation revealed better results for the group receiving the Wobenzym N preparation. The differences between the two groups were significant with respect to three important inflammation markers: C–reaction protein (see Chapter 10 for information on this important marker of overall body inflammation); α1–trypsin; and the erythrocyte sedimentation rate. The changes in general state of health (e.g., dysphagia [difficulty in swallowing] and swelling of the lymph nodes) and all objective variables of wound healing were clear–cut evidence of the clear superiority of Wobenzym N therapy.

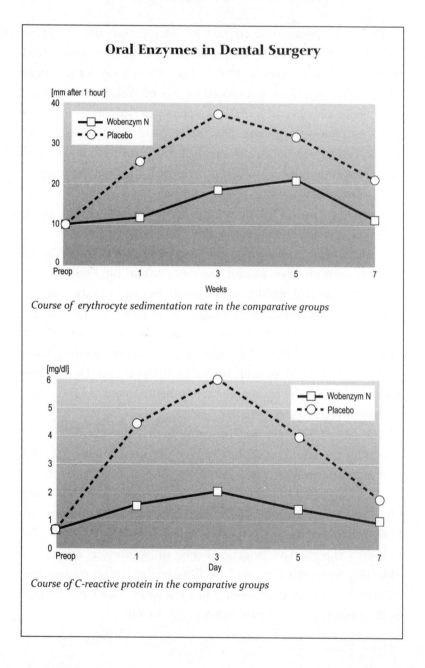

Course of erythrocyte sedimentation rate in the comparative groups

Course of C-reactive protein in the comparative groups

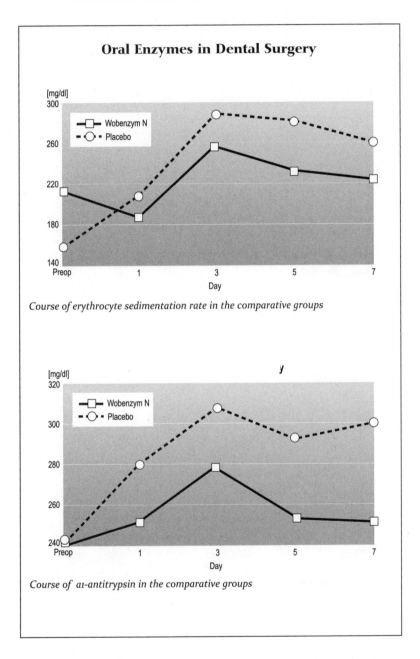

Oral Enzymes in Dental Surgery

Course of erythrocyte sedimentation rate in the comparative groups

Course of a1-antitrypsin in the comparative groups

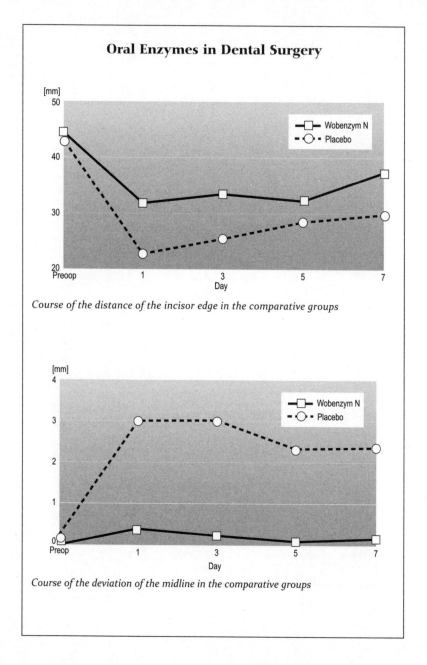

Course of the distance of the incisor edge in the comparative groups

Course of the deviation of the midline in the comparative groups

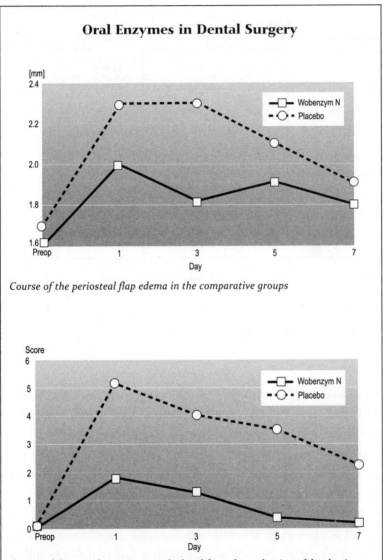

Oral Enzymes in Dental Surgery

Course of the periosteal flap edema in the comparative groups

Course of the cumulative scores, calculated from the evaluation of dysphagia as well as palpable and painful swelling in the lymph nodes in the preparation group in comparison with that of the control group

Oral Enzymes in Dental Surgery							
	Wobenzym®N Preparation				Placebo		
	1st day		7th day		1st day		7th day	
	n	%	n	%	n	%	n	%
(1) No signs of irritation	23	63.9	34	94.4	23	52.3	29	65.9
(2) Redness	8	22.2	1	2.8	9	20.5	6	13.6
(3) Purulence	2	5.6	-	-	2	4.6	-	-
(4) Hematoma	1	2.8	-	-	4	9.1	2	4.6
(5) Seroma	1	2.8	-	-	4	9.1	5	11.4
(6) Hematoma and sermoma	-	-	-	-	1	2.3	1	2.3
Not indicated	1	2.8	1	2.8	1	2.8	1	2.3
Total	36	100.0	35	100.0	44	100.0	44	100.0
Mean value	1.54		1.03*		2.9		1.88	

* significantly better than in the placebo group

Evaluation of wound healing in the preparation and control groups

Proctology

Proctology is the branch of medicine dealing with the rectum and anus. Aside from a few exceptions, anal wounds generally heal by secondary intention. Local therapy consists of sitz baths and the support of wound cleansing with chains of complex sugars derived from sucrose called dextran polymers. Regular digital palpation hinders the development of superficial adhesions and pocketing. Since the anal region is very sensitive to pain, the use of analgesics is generally unavoidable. Regulation of bowel movements must be ensured during the first two weeks following surgery. Wobenzym N can be extremely useful in helping persons who must undergo surgery for such problems, including hemorrhoids, anal fissures, and spreading abscesses within the anus that can erode the tissue and which are known medically as anal fistulas.

Using a topical preparation of Wobenzym N, Drs. Chappa–Alvarez and Werk achieved a substantially more rapid healing rate following proctological operations, as they reported in 1979 in *Proktologie.*[70] Thirty patients in two groups of 15 persons each took part in this study. All patients were treated conventionally, and one group received Wobenzym N ointment locally in addition. Pain, edema, secretion, hemorrhage and scar formation served as evaluation criteria for the progress of healing during the treatment period, which lasted an average of 15 days. The investigators objectified the clinical findings as far as possible by histological examination.

Within only a few days, the number of leukocytes (white blood cells) in the surgical wound increased threefold in patients treated with enzymes, a sign of excellent, non–infectious wound healing.

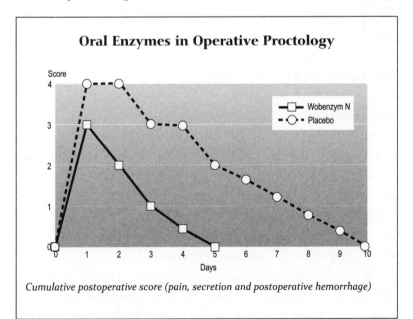

Oral Enzymes in Operative Proctology

Cumulative postoperative score (pain, secretion and postoperative hemorrhage)

As an indicator of beginning granulation (remodeling of the wound), levels of large white blood cells called monocytes that are formed in the bone marrow increased by 100%. Aside from the rate of healing, which was 40% faster in the group receiving the topical Wobenzym N, the group receiving this preparation also demonstrated substantially less pain.

The clinical complaints disappeared completely after only 40 to 50 days. The persistence of symptoms lasted substantially longer in the control group–for up to 100 days.

Lower Extremity Bypass Surgery

Wobenzym N may be critical to anyone who must undergo heart bypass surgery. Knowing that the antiedema and anti-inflammatory characteristics of Wobenzym N have been strongly verified for various surgeries prompted Dr. H.-D. Rahn to examine the use of Wobenzym N for vascular reconstructive surgery of the lower extremities. Dr. Rahn examined its efficacy in a clinical, placebo–controlled, double–blind study on 80 patients who were undergoing heart bypass surgery.[71]

Patients taking part in the study all had stage IIB to IV arterial occlusion or occlusive arterial disease, necessitating treatment of the afflicted leg with an artificial or vein bypass. In this procedure, an incision is made in one or both of the legs and length of vein is removed. Meanwhile, another incision is made down the center of the chest and the rib cage is opened to expose the heart. The surgeon then uses the vein the from the leg to make one or more grafts to bypass the blockages in the coronary artery and so restore the blood flow to normal.

Obviously, recovery is relatively extended and may require several days in intensive care with attention to be paid both to the condition of the heart as well as the leg or legs. (In this study, patients

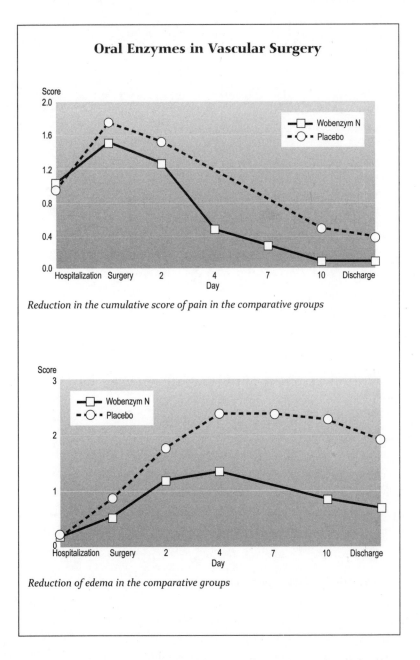

Reduction in the cumulative score of pain in the comparative groups

Reduction of edema in the comparative groups

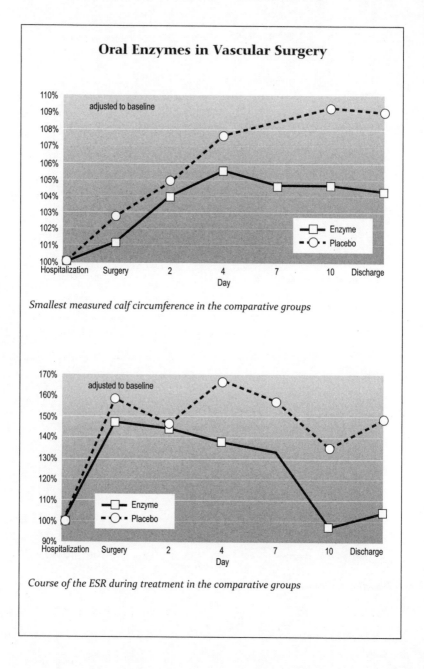

Smballest measured calf circumference in the comparative groups

Course of the ESR during treatment in the comparative groups

who had taken non-steroidal antirheumatic agents within the last three preoperative days were excluded from the study.) Assignment of patients to the two groups of 40 patients was at random.

Three days prior to surgery, the patients of the preparation and control groups began taking one measuring spoon of granulated Wobenzym N or an equal amount of granulated placebo three times daily. The therapy was continued during the entire in-hospital period up to 14 days.

Assessment of treatment efficacy was based on measurements of the circumference of the afflicted leg at three defined positions, the extent of edema and the cumulative pain score. The other clinical parameters (e.g., local temperature, wound healing) as well as the length of hospitalization were recognized as additional criteria for evaluation. Laboratory data included ESR, white blood cell and platelet counts, Quick's time and antithrombin III. Enzyme therapy resulted in a significantly better treatment outcome with respect to these main and additional criteria. Aside from ESR, the differences in laboratory data were not substantial.

Traumatology

In 1972, Dr. A.R. Carillo and co-investigators examined the efficacy of Wobenzym in 100 patients with various injuries or burns in order to verify the numerous positive reports and obtain an idea of the possibilities for applying systemic oral enzymes.[72]

Ten to twenty coated Wobenzym N tablets were prescribed daily in addition to the necessary conservative or surgical therapeutic measures. The average duration of treatment with enzymes was six days.

Even though Wobenzym N has modulating properties on the body's blood flow, the Carillo team noted no increased risk of hem-

Oral Enzymes in Traumatology

Diagnosis	Number of cases	very good	good	moderate	poor
Sprains	18	15	3	–	–
Contusions	22	21	1	–	–
Fractures and multiple injuries	20	19	1	–	–
Phlebitis and varicose edema	8	7	–	1	–
Neuritis	2	2	–	–	–
Unspecified arthritis	8	3	1	3	1
Wounds, felons, tendosynovitis	12	11	1	–	–
Burns	4	3	1	–	–
Hematomas (longer than 48 h)	6	1	1	3	1
Total	**100**	**82**	**9**	**7**	**2**

Results of therapy differentiated by nosological entities

orrhage. Dr. Carillo evaluated the fibrinolytic action of the enzyme preparation as being positive in every respect. The healing of injuries and burns was substantially accelerated with Wobenzym N.

Only four patients complained of slight gastric intolerance. The symptoms resolved after simply increasing the time between individual doses.

In summary, Dr. Carillo found that Wobenzym N has a rapid and convincing anti-inflammatory action which substantially accelerates the rate of healing for patients undergoing surgery for trauma and burns.

Pre- and Postoperative Enzyme Therapy for Fracture Reduction

Wobenzym N is also key for improving the outcome of surgery for fractures and dislocations. In the case of surgical fracture, for example, reduction of the fractured region requires optimal preparation–which always includes the rapid and efficient treatment of posttraumatic edema and hematoma. Systemic oral enzymes can be extremely beneficial in such surgeries.

The efficacy of preoperatively initiated enzyme therapy was verified by Drs. H.-D. Rahn and M. Kilic in a placebo–controlled, double–blind study of 120 patients requiring operative fracture reduction that was published in 1990 in *Allgenmeinarzt*.[73, 74]

Both study groups of 60 patients each began by taking ten coated tablets of Wobenzym N or placebo three times daily prior to surgery. Relief of pain and reduction of the edema were substantially better in the Wobenzym N group after only three days. This significant difference between the two comparative groups continued postoperatively. An added bonus that should be emphasized is that the patients on oral enzymes were able to leave the hospital earlier!

With the goal of verifying the antiedema effects of Wobenzym N more exactly, Dr. Schwinger performed an open, prospective, randomized clinical study on parallel groups. The efficacy and tolerability of Wobenzym N was compared with that of aescin, a powerful healing extract from the horse chestnut seed.

Extent of Fracture Associated Edema

	Wobenzym˚N	Placebo
Preoperative		
Day of admission	100%	100%
Third day prior to surgery	53%	71%
Day of surgery	21%	57%
Postoperative		
1st postoperative day	100%	100%
5th postoperative day	42%	42%
7th postoperative day	11%	17%

Extent of edema with respect to the initial pre- and postoperative findings

Intensity of Pre– and Postoperative Pain

	Wobenzym°N	Placebo
Preoperative		
Day of admission	100%	100%
Third day prior to surgery	40%	50%
Day of surgery	27%	41%
Postoperative		
1st postoperative day	100%	100%
5th postoperative day	29%	34%
7th postoperative day	9%	20%

Extent of pain intensity with respect to the initial pre- and postoperative findings

Effect of Wobenzym® versus Placebo on Hospital Stay

Preoperative Wobenzym®N	19.3 days
Preoperative placebo	22.6 days
Postoperative Wobenzym®N	19.5 days
Postoperative placebo	22.3 days
Pre- and postoperative Wobenzym®N	17.7 days
Pre- and postoperative placebo	24.1 days

Hospital stay

Fifty–nine patients with injuries of the knees or ankle joints requiring surgical treatment took part in this study. Depending on the group assignment, 29 patients received five coated Wobenzym N tablets three times daily and 30 patients two coated tablets of aescin three times daily. The duration of therapy was ten days. The groups were matched for age, sex, edema, joint effusion, inflammation, pain, ability to raise the extended leg, and their cumulative pain scores.

The circumference of the joint and the pain score were established as the main inflammatory criteria for the study.

Additional criteria were further clinical and laboratory data and the use of analgesics.

Although aescin is another excellent natural medicine, it must be said that, all in all, the joint swelling in the enzyme group diminished to a greater extent. The substantial reduction in the swelling of the ankle joint was statistically significant. The drop in pain scores was nearly equal for both groups, although it must be mentioned that the aescin group required substantially greater amounts of analgesics. No statistically significant differences were seen between the therapy with Wobenzym N versus aescin for any of the other criteria examined.[75]

Knee Surgery (Meniscectomy and Arthroscopic)

Another type of knee surgery is meniscectomy, in which a specific type of cartilage is removed. A double-blind study was conducted on 80 patients who had to undergo total meniscectomy. Whereas 40 patients were treated with enzymes postoperatively, the other 40 test subjects received a placebo. The patients were instructed to take 30 coated tablets of Wobenzym N or the dummy pills daily. The duration of therapy was seven days for both groups. Edema, swelling, inflammation, pain and limitation of mobility were examined to evaluate the efficiency of the therapy. The symptom complex responded significantly better to the postoperative administration of Wobenzym N. It was possible to mobilize the patients earlier to restore the mobility of the knee joint.[76, 77]

Arthroscopic operations on the knee joint have also become well established in recent years, the technique being superior to open surgery. It therefore appeared relevant to examine the efficacy of Wobenzym N especially in arthroscopic meniscectomies–in a further clinical, placebo-controlled,

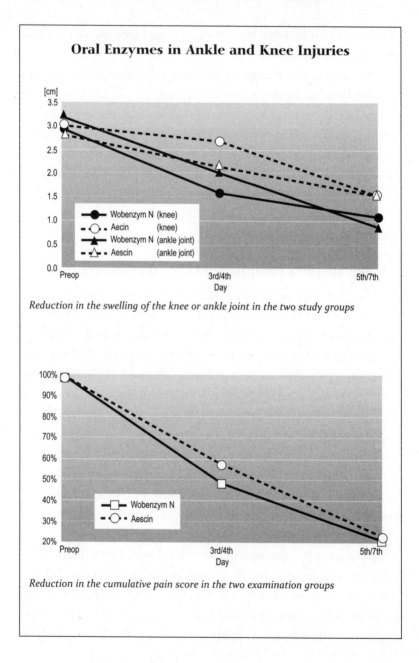

Oral Enzymes in Ankle and Knee Injuries

Reduction in the swelling of the knee or ankle joint in the two study groups

Reduction in the cumulative pain score in the two examination groups

double-blind study, 80 patients with 40 patients each in the enzyme preparation and placebo groups.[78] The test subjects received Wobenzym N for an average of nine days. The patient groups were matched with respect to age, sex, height, weight and severity of the injury. The statistical evaluation was based on a defined cumulative score consisting of data on edema, pain and limitation of mobility. Additionally assessed was improvement of further clinical parameters and the duration of the hospital stay. The cumulative scores of the Wobenzym N group dropped significantly faster and more substantially, confirming clinical effectiveness.

Recent Studies

Most recently researchers at the Stavropol State Medical Academy, Pediatric Surgery department, reported in the December 2009 issue of the *European Journal of Pediatric Surgery* that polyenzyme therapy could help after undergoing abdominal surgery by reducing extracellular growth factors causing scarring or what are known as adhesion. Said the researchers, "The mean adhesion grades of the enzyme group were significantly lower than in the control group."

Yet another recent study also found very favorable results. Reporting in the May–June 2009 issue of *Vopr Kurortol Fizioter Lech Fiz Kult* in a Russian language article, researchers tested Wobenzym N on 393 patients with fractured long bones (humeral, radial/ulnar, femoral, crural) admitted to the Orthopedic Department of the Stavropol Regional Children's Clinical Hospital and the Rehabilitation Centre for Handicapped Children and Adolescents. Rehabilitation was performed in three consecutive stages, viz. immobilization, functional recovery and training. The proposed approach ensured rather fast functional recovery of the affected extremity even in cases with compound fractures. The rehabilitation program included polyenzyme therapy with Wobenzym N during three to four weeks after injury or surgical repositioning of bone fragments. "Pain and edema syndromes resolved twice as fast as after traditional treatment. The use of this program… improved the quality of life in children with fractures of long tubular bones."

Additionally, researchers report in the November–December 2006 issue of *Vestn Oftalmol* that systemic enzyme therapy helps children with fractures of the orbital wall. Wobenzym N was used in 26 children with lower orbital wall fractures as monotherapy in early periods (on days 1 to 7) after brain injury to improve healing conditions and to minimize the formation of scar tissues in the fractural area. A control group comprised 24 patients who received systemic dehydration and vessel–strengthening therapy. Systemic enzyme therapy reduced the inflammatory manifestations of injury, prevented complications, and substantially decreased the number of patients having indications for surgical plastic repair of the orbital wall, as compared with the control group.

The Bottom Line

Hundreds of published scientific studies and our own clinical reports have shown that systemic oral enzymes act to quickly reduce inflammation, swelling, and internal bleeding, all of which are extremely important to control following surgery. What's more, enzymes are extremely safe, especially compared to other anti–inflammatory medical drugs that were designed for this purpose.

Doctors recognize that surgery produces edema, inflammation and excessive fibrinolytic activity, all of which must be treated to insure the patient's rapid recovery. Because Wobenzym N provides a comprehensive therapeutic effect in all of these areas of need and without complications, it is considered as pre- and post-operative frontline therapy throughout Europe. It should be in America, too.

Wobenzym N has been used successfully throughout Europe for over 20 years in surgery and traumatology, and has been described in numerous published reports and case histories.

Among its extremely well documented uses is the prevention and treatment of edema and inflammation in operative dental procedures; proctological operations; surgery to repair fracture of the upper and lower leg; arthroscopic knee surgery; vascular reconstructive surgery of the lower legs; and burns.[79, 80]

How to Use Wobenzym N
if You're Undergoing Surgery

Systemic enzymes are NOT a drug. Within the US regulatory framework, they should not be touted to treat, cure or diagnose disease. I see these powerful natural molecules as agents that support healthy functions in the body and strengthen these. With this in mind, always inform your physician before

---

High Dosages vs. Median Dosages
for Acute Trauma and Surgery

In cases of acute trauma, seek qualified professional help from an emergency room physician or other qualified health professional. Upon stabilization, an initial dose of ten tablets three times daily is advisable in acute cases of trauma in contrast to the usual maintenance dose of two to three coated tablets three times daily.[81]

beginning use of systemic enzymes prior to surgery. If there is any contraindication for enzyme therapy, it is in patients who are at risk of post-operative hemorrhage because of blood coagulation deficiency, heavy bleeders, hyperfibrinolysis, and severe liver cirrhosis or among patients who must undergo surgery in which there may be extreme loss of blood. However, enzyme therapy can be used with doctor's knowledge after other appropriate surgeries, as detailed in this chapter. Start your use two to three days before surgery. The recommended dosage before surgery is ten tablets three times a day 30 to 45 minutes before meals.

8

Systemic Oral Enzymes and Soft-tissue Injuries

Another important application where systemic oral enzymes equal or outperform the benefits to be arrived from NSAIDs is in the area of soft tissue injuries–the most common kinds of injuries people suffer. They affect connective and other "soft" tissues rather than the bones, and often involve extreme inflammation, redness and swelling as well as pain. Patients are often able to take care of themselves but this also means a safe, efficient, self-applied therapy with few adverse effects is all the more important, since they will be predominantly self-medicating.

In a double-blind, randomized parallel group study, researchers examined the effectiveness and tolerance of Wobenzym N in soft-tissue injuries sustained in athletics.[82] The study included 44 patients with various types of injuries. Twenty-two patients each took Wobenzym N or placebo. The median length of therapy was 11 days. The lessening of pain and in the diameter of hematomas was taken as the primary criteria for statistical evaluation.

The results of the study provided impressive evidence that pain and hematomas due to injury can be reduced significantly and more rapidly with Wobenzym N. The advantage of enzyme therapy was also reflected in the reduced need for analgesics and the earlier mobilization in the group taking the enzyme mixture. As a result the rate of absence due to injury was sub-stantially shorter.

Wobenzym N and Reabsorption of Hematomas

Hematomas are masses of blood, caused by the breakage of ves-sels. These injuries can cause significant disturbances of the heal-ing process. An important aspect in treating sports and other injuries is reducing their negative effects.

The influence of enzymes on the re-absorption of hematomas due to trauma and the reduction in the pain they cause was studied in a randomized, controlled, double-blind study based on artificial hematomas. (The researchers collected blood from the cubital vein of 100 voluntary test subjects and injected it sub-cutaneously into the inner surface of the opposite arm.) The hematoma which developed was comparable to a normal hematoma caused by trauma.

One half of the test subjects took either Wobenzym N or placebo for one week. Evaluation was based on swelling, sensa-tion of tension, and pain on pressure. Absorption of the hematoma was 12 percent faster when the oral enzyme mixture was taken. The cumulative value and the duration of pain on pressure in the enzyme group was about 45 percent less than that in the placebo group.

9
Healing Sports Injuries Naturally

Another important application of systemic oral enzymes is with sports injuries. Indeed, systemic oral enzymes are probably far superior to conventional painkillers for athletes at all levels of competition, including weekend warriors, occasional joggers and other recreational participants.

Americans are more aware than ever before of the positive effects of exercise and proper nutrition. The drastic increase of recreational sports and fitness during the last quarter century is a lifestyle revolution.

Exercise is one of the most important things people can do to create great physical and mental health. Exercise not only helps persons to lose weight, control food cravings, reduce the risk of diabetes, heart and circulatory disease and cancer. Exercise also helps the body to create feel-good endorphins, tiny neuropeptides comprised of amino acids that resemble opiates and that are released by the brain in response to stress or trauma, reacting with the brain's opiate receptors to reduce the sensation of pain; fortunately, their effects carry over long after our exercise is finished, fostering a positive mental outlook on life.

This fitness boom, however, has a downside: sports injuries are becoming increasingly prevalent as more and more health conscious people start to exercise daily. What's more, too many athletes at all levels are turning to drugs, such as over-the-counter or prescription medications, to overcome their injuries and in an attempt to excel at their athletic endeavors. As a physician and educator, who have worked with some of the world's greatest champions, we are here to say that today's new breed of championship athlete can succeed without drugs, and that we are one-hundred percent for creating champions—and equally opposed to the indiscriminate and proliferating use of street and potentially toxic medical drugs in conjunction with sports.

Every year, millions of athletes of all ages suffer debilitating injuries. They usually end up taking pain killers such as aspirin or other over-the-counter preparations known as non-steroidal anti-inflammatory drugs. These formulas may quench the pain, but they do nothing to initiate the healing process and their long-term use poses significant complications.

We have a better way to heal sport injuries.

To focus on one country—the Czech Republic—this all-natural supplement is one of the keys to success for athletes such as world champion record holders Jan Zelezny in the javelin and Daniela Bartová in the pole vault. It is the key training aid used by Olympic decathlete champion Robert Zmelik, as well as fellow world champion Tomás Dvoräk; and triple jump world champion Sarka Kazpárková. In professional tennis, Martina Hingis, who uses this all-natural performance and training aid, has been ranked number one or two in the Women's Tennis Association.

Moving elsewhere in the world, Ukraine boxer Oleg Kiriukhin, who was a bronze medallist in the 1996 Olympic Games in Atlanta, uses this formula daily to aid his training and heal his body faster.

Closer to home, the formula is used by European hockey stars Jaromir Jagr of the National Hockey League's Pittsburgh Penguins;

Zikamind Pullfy of the New York Islanders; and Peter Bondra of the Washington Capitals.

The list could go on and on.

Perhaps one other story will illustrate the importance of this supplement to athletic performance and training. It has long been know that within the entire Soviet block, the best sport scientists were found in East Germany. After all, this tiny, racially and ethnically homogenous nation with its limited gene pool and population of only about seventeen million dominated so many Olympic events throughout the 1960s through the 1980s.

The East German sports scientists and doctors, it was well known, were highly advanced in developing performance and training regimens, including methods for the deplorable masking of the doping of their champion athletes. The East Germans were, in fact, the first country to systematically use androsteinedione and other banned androgens.

In 1984, when the Olympic Games came to the Balkans for the first time, although the Soviet Union would finish the Sarajevo Games with the most medals, 25, it was the East Germans who would strike gold the most, with individuals and teams finishing first in ski jumping, women's figure skating, women's speedskating, women's luge, and the two-man and four-man bobsled—for a total of nine gold medals.

Christa Rothenburger (East Germany) set an Olympic record in her gold medal performance in the women's 500 meter speedskating competition. Second place finisher Karin Enke, also from East Germany, captured the gold in both the 1,000 and 1,500 meter race. Andrea Schone completed the East German sweep of the women's speedskating events with a gold medal in the 3,000 meters. East German women won 11 of 13 gold medals in swimming at both the 1976 and 1980 Olympics.

Unfortunately, recent studies have revealed that between 6,000 and 10,000 athletes were covered by a systematic doping program that operated in the former Communist country. And, yet, there were also many advances in natural medicine within the East German sport training regimen. The East German athletes still needed to be able to recover more quickly from their training as well as injuries. They needed a formula to quell inflammation quickly and safely.

This is where our natural supplement comes into play. For a very long time, Mucos Pharma GmbH, the German manufacturer of systemic oral enzyme preparations, was receiving orders for large amounts of their famous enzyme formula, Wobenzym N, from various agents in Vienna and other European cities. Of course, as the orders came in, hundreds of thousands of Wobenzym N tablets would be promptly shipped, it was thought, to be used in medical settings such as hospitals and clinics. Little did Mucos Pharma realize how its premiere enzyme formula was really being used . . .

In 1989, the Berlin Wall came down and Germany was on its pathway to reunification. Now that travel through Checkpoint Charley was once again legal, Mucos Pharma scientists visited hospitals in the former East Germany, expecting to see large amounts of Wobenzym N–yet, they saw none! The mystery remained.

One night in the mid-1990s scientists from Mucos Pharma GmbH were at a dinner where one of the guests was the former head of the East German Physical Culture Institute. It was during the social hour that the former East German administrator admitted that it had been they who were purchasing the Wobenzym N tablets through various middlemen, smuggling it into East Germany, and that their athletes used Wobenzym N–a completely legal substance–in very large amounts to lower the effects of training and especially to safely and naturally stave off inflammation, redness and swelling.

The East German official explained that whenever athletes train, they will always incur microtrauma to the tendons and ligaments and place stress on the joint matrix. Wobenzym N was the perfect answer to maintain healthy joint function and range of motion. The androgens were, of course, important, but perfectly useless to an athlete beset by injury. If the East German athletes could moderate their inflammation, they could maintain full strength and range of motion. He also mentioned unpublished data that Wobenzym N was in itself a perfectly natural and highly effective anabolic aid for building strength, muscle, and endurance. Finally, the mystery behind the huge orders for Wobenzym N was revealed.

But now, the task at end was even more challenging: inform athletes worldwide about this legal, acceptable, ethical, safe and proven performance aid that the East Germans also used– Wobenzym N systemic oral enzymes.

Hundreds of published scientific studies and European doctors' own clinical experience have shown that enzymes act to quickly reduce inflammation, swelling, and internal bleeding, all of which are extremely important to control following surgery. What's more, enzymes are extremely safe, especially compared to other anti–inflammatory medical drugs that were designed for this purpose.

Systemic Oral Enzymes and Sports Injuries: Worth Their Weight in Olympic Gold

Hermann Maier

Shiga Kogen, Japan. Picabo Street singing "The Star-Spangled Banner" with a gold medal around her neck. Alberto Tomba lying in the snow, grabbing his sore back. Katja Seizinger leaping off the victory stand. These are some of the images that we will longer remember when we think back on the 1998 Winter Olympic Games. And then there was Austrian alpine skier Hermann Maier.

Despite days of snow, rain, fog and wind that caused maddening delays and scheduling nightmares, the Alpine skiing events provided some of the most compelling images of the Nagano Games.

None, though, could match the horrifying sight of Maier flying sideways through the air and crashing through two safety nets. The press and critics were certain his Olympic saga and gold medal quest ended with that terrifying crash. Yet, Maier went on to return from the bruises, swelling, redness, tenderness and acute pain, both physical and mental, of his awful tumble to win two gold medals within the next six days. Maier's crash indeed provided one of the lasting images from the Games.

But what few know about Hermann Maier is that, besides his intense competitor's drive, the Austrian champion was using a very special, scientifically formulated enzyme formula. This formula, now available in the United States, is the leading sports injury medicine in the world. It is only just now being discovered by our American athletes. It was this formula that Maier's own doctor has publicly stated helped his star patient overcome his terrible injuries and aided tremendously in stimulating the healing process that enabled him to return to action quickly.

According to Maier's doctor, his daily use of Wobenzym N systemic oral enzymes, long before the accident, was, in fact, one of the principal reasons he suffered no lasting serious injury during his terrible free fall down the rugged mountainous slope. In fact, the Austrian and German Winter Olympic teams ordered more than one million pills of this natural medicine for the 1998 Olympics. Why? Because they want to win, and systemic oral enzymes provide them with a drug-free edge over the competition.

Bobbi Gale Bensman

If you want to talk about a tough sport that is sure to make for sore and inflamed muscles, that sport would have to be rock climbing and bouldering. It's man vs. rock. Or, in the case of Bobbi Gale Bensman, woman vs. rock.

Nationally ranked among the top three rock climbers from 1987 to 1995 and a winner of more than 20 national competitions, Bensman knows all about sports injuries and soreness. She swears by systemic oral enzymes.

"Being a competitive and intense athlete, I think that systemic oral enzymes are essential to take daily," she says. "Systemic oral enzymes are remarkable for enhancing my energy levels and healing from injuries. When I am run down or have sprains, tendon or joint problems, I'll increase my dosage and come back even quicker."

"I just took a trip to Australia in April and May," she continues. "I was hiking down a really steep hill and twisted my ankle. I had run out of my enzymes and the injury lasted for a month. When I arrived home, the first thing I did was to start taking five tablets on an empty stomach two to three times a day. Once I was using enzymes, the swelling and soreness disappeared within a few days. Let me tell you from my own personal experience:

enzymes work better than ibuprofen and without side effects, which is important to a competitive athlete like me.

"But there are a lot of other reasons I take systemic oral enzymes daily. The formula is great for digestion and enhancing my resistance to colds and the flu. Systemic oral enzymes are just a great product all around for making your body work better."

Stefi Graf

On June 12, 1997, in an attempt to quell growing expectations of a quick recovery after undergoing knee surgery in Vienna, tennis star Stefi Graf announced to the world press that she would certainly miss Wimbledon and the U.S. Open. Even the German Sunday newspaper *Welt Am Sonntag* hinted that there was no guarantee she would resume her career following her knee operation in Vienna.

But the former world number one tennis player and twenty-one times Grand Slam champion had a secret tool to help her recover after the two-hour operation on her left knee at an undisclosed hospital in the Austrian capital. Her secret? A skilled surgeon and, as her own personal physician personally stated, many of his top athletes regularly use Wobenzym N systemic oral enzymes. Less than a year later, Graf was competing again and winning.

Throughout the world today, athletes, from weekend warriors to Olympic gold medallists, have discovered the secret of systemic oral enzymes. German figure skating Olympian Katarina Witt and tennis start Boris Becker, to name a few, are thought to use the Wobenzym N systemic oral enzyme system—but there are many more athletes who are also champions in sports as diverse as track and field, hockey, skiing, boxing, karate, soccer and American football, who are also using systemic oral enzymes to excel and reach their very peak of fitness and competitiveness.

Do these championship athletes and weekend warriors know something about keeping healthy and avoiding sports injuries that other injury-riddled athletes have yet to learn?

What is this secret, then? What are these special enzymes? Are they approved for use by international sport governing bodies? Are they a food? Are they a drug? Nutritional supplement? Are they proven with medical studies? What can they do for elite athletes? What can they do to help weekend warriors? Can they benefit children and high school athletes? How can they help you, whether you are an elite athlete, competing in the masters class or a collegiate, high school or junior level athlete? What if you are simply a walker or work-out daily on your treadmill and want to stay healthy and in shape? Can systemic oral enzymes help you to stay healthy and fit without requiring toxic prescription medications and possibly other even less safe drugs?

Bottom Line

You can turn on the amazing healing powers in your own body and initiate dramatic improvements in your health if you are suffering from sports injuries by following our comprehensive ten point program. It consists of the following elements:

- ❖ Proper diet.
- ❖ Daily use of systemic oral enzymes.
- ❖ Aerobic and conditioning exercise.
- ❖ Stretching.
- ❖ Weight loss, if necessary.
- ❖ Avoiding repetitive motion.
- ❖ Using biomechanics and ergonomics.
- ❖ Alleviating stress.
- ❖ Maintaining a positive outlook on life–even in the face of adverse circumstances such as painful joints.

❖ Maintaining a balanced sensible approach to training and competition and never giving up.

You can experience a significant improvement in your health if you are suffering from any degenerative or acute sports injury. We're here to coax, persuade, and motivate you into action to get your quest for the ultimate in sports back on track by our ten point healing program, and especially the use of drug-free systemic oral enzymes.

Two Major Types of Sport Injuries

On a whole there are two main types of sports injuries: those from overuse and those that are acute.

Overuse Injuries

Overuse injuries are characteristic of an accumulation of repetitive trauma to the tissues of the body. Most activities that cause these injuries involve prolonged repetitive movement of large muscle groups. Sometimes the problem is more mental than physical.

Sports are a great outlet for emotions that build-up in us, but they should not become an obsession, and one area to which athletes must be sensitized is to interactions between mind and emotion. Chronic use injuries often are a telltale sign of over-training with subsequent chronic use or overuse injuries. If you're overtraining, you won't be as effective an athlete. Athletes should recognize that they will perform best when they balance training with other important areas of life. Still, the pursuit of excellence requires tireless training, and tennis or pitcher's elbow, shin splints, hip pointers, and other chronic overuse injuries are likely to become part of the elite athlete's life. Systemic oral enzymes are especially beneficial in reducing the inflammation and soreness, allowing for quicker recovery.

Acute Injuries

On the other hand, an acute injury occurs from one incident. These injuries are often seen in contact sports and could be thought of as "traditional injuries." Sprains, strains, bruises and breaks all fall into this category. There are two sub-types of acute injuries: those to the soft tissues and those to the bones or skeletal injuries.

—Soft Tissue Injuries

About 95 percent of sports injuries are due to minor trauma involving soft tissue injuries–sprains, strains (muscle pulls), contusions, bruises, and cuts or abrasions. The patients are often able to take of themselves. A safe and efficient therapy with few adverse effects is all the more mandatory. Systemic oral enzymes are probably the athlete's greatest healing friend when it comes to soft tissue injuries because there is no toxicity and, as a result, the athlete can self-medicate without fear of long-term complications, while achieving both pain relief and stimulating healing.

Sprains. About one-third of all sports injuries are classified as sprains, defined as a *partial or complete tear of a ligament,* which is the tough band of fibrous connective tissue that connects the ends of bones and stabilizes the joint. Symptoms include the feeling that a joint is "loose" or unstable; an inability to bear weight because of pain; loss of motion; the sound or feeling of a "pop" or "snap" when the injury occurred, and swelling.

Strains. A strain is a *partial or complete tear of a muscle or tendon.* Muscle tissue is made up of cells that contract and make the body move. A tendon consists of tough connective tissue that attaches muscles to bones.

Contusions. The most common sports injury is a contusion or *bruise.* Bruises result when a blunt injury causes underlying bleeding in a muscle or other soft tissues. Treatment for soft tissue injuries usually consists of rest, applying ice, wrapping with elastic bandages (compression), and elevating the injured arm, hand, leg or foot. Hematomas, or leakage of blood, may develop.

Spinal cord injuries. Although rare in sports, 10 percent of all spinal injuries occur during sports, primarily diving, surfing and football. Participants in contact sports can minimize the risk of minor neck spinal injuries such as sprains and pinched nerves by doing exercises to strengthen their neck muscles.

—Skeletal Injuries

A sudden, violent collision with another player, an accident with sports equipment, or a severe fall can cause skeletal injuries in the growing athlete, including fractures. Skeletal injuries occur far less frequently than soft tissue injuries.

Fractures constitute a low five to six percent of all sports injuries. Most of these breaks occur in the arms and legs. Rarely are the spine and skull fractured.

Stress fractures frequently occur because of continuing overuse of a joint. The main symptom of a stress fracture is pain. The most frequent places stress fractures occur are the tibia (the larger leg bone below the knee), fibula (the outer and thinner leg bone below the knee), and foot.

How Systemic Oral Enzymes Accelerate Healing of Sports Injuries

"Rubor et tumor cum calore et dolore." In the first century A.D., Celsus pretty much summed up the classical signs of inflammation: redness, swelling, heat and pain. He neglected to mention loss of function, a seat on the sidelines, and the intense frustration that all benched athletes experience.

After an injury, a sequence of events is set in motion at the cellular and biochemical levels that results in resolution. In general, the healing response can be divided into three major portions or phases: inflammation, repair, and remodeling. In each of these phases enzymes can help to heal the body quickly and safely.

How Enzymes Work

Immediately after injury, acute vasoconstriction lasts for a few minutes until a number of chemical mediators exert their effects. One such chemical mediator is called bradykinin. It is a hormone that dilates blood vessels and increase capillary permeability, allowing for the transport of additional healing agents. Meanwhile, leukocytes initiate movement of additional white blood cells to the injured area to continue getting rid of damaged and dying tissue and prevent infection. This increased presence of white blood cells causes release of massive amounts of additional proinflammatory mediators and leads to expression of the clinical signs of inflammation. Inflammation induces edema.

Unless the healing process is optimized, subacute inflammation may linger for weeks or months.

Most sport injuries, no matter how serious, involve redness, inflammation and swelling and require both immediate and long-term treatment. Systemic oral enzymes are superior for treatment because they directly influence each of the phases of sports injuries without complications associated typically with the NSAID class of drugs that are typically prescribed.

Wobenzym N, the world's leading enzyme formula, also contains rutin, a bioflavonoid, which normalizes damaged vessels and helps to encourage transportation of the body's own defensive substances required for healing to the site of inflammation.

Systemic oral enzymes allow the body to enter the repair and remodeling phases of sports injuries more quickly than you ever imagined.

Repair
The second phase of healing sports injuries is the repair phase. The repair phase is characterized by cell growth and production of extracellular matrix (collagen and proteoglycans). During this phase, enzymes help by reducing scarring or sclerosis.

Remodeling
The third phase is called remodeling (maturation) which occurs about 14 days after the injury. Granulation tissues shift from Type II to Type I collage, and collagen synthetic activity approaches normal turnover. Systemic oral enzymes enable the body to enter the remodeling phase more quickly, as shown in more than one dozen studies in which injured athletes given Wobenzym N have been able to return to action much more quickly than athletes given typical NSAIDs or placebo.

Studies that Support Natural Healing of Sports Injuries with Systemic Oral Enzymes

In almost all sports injuries, if you are injured, initial therapy should consist of cooling, compression, elevation and rest.

Typically, a doctor might prescribe aspirin, ibuprofen, or another type of pain killer, usually known as a non–steroidal anti-inflammatory drug (NSAID), for sports and exercise injuries, particularly when there is inflammation. NSAIDs do, in fact, work well for quickly relieving pain and inflammation, and people generally can safely use NSAIDs for up to a few days. *But what happens next is key to whether your injury will linger or quickly heal.*

We believe in providing patients with the safest, most effective treatment strategies for sports injuries. We also believe that sports should be drug-free. Wobenzym® N is not only safer than ibuprofen and other similar drugs for long-term use, it's often more effective and its use is approved by all major sports governing bodies.

Hundreds of published scientific studies and our own clinical experience have shown that enzymes act to quickly reduce inflammation, swelling, and internal bleeding, all of which are extremely important to control following injury. What's more, enzymes are extremely safe, especially compared to other anti-inflammatory medical drugs that were designed for this purpose.

Throughout Europe, sports medicine doctors have discovered a natural, safer pathway for healing sports and exercise-related injuries. For athletes with both acute and chronic injuries, a quality enzyme mixture is by far the superior choice both for reducing inflammation and safety.

Enzymes are one of the most powerful, yet little known healing secrets now available to American consumers who are concerned with inflammation and sports injuries. We often recommend enzymes over any other type of pain reliever because they work so well and are very safe.

Studies that Validate Enzymes for Sports Injuries

It is important to note that virtually all of the sport injury studies done on enzymes were sponsored by Mucos Pharma GmbH, of Germany, producer of the world famous Wobenzym N systemic oral enzyme formula. Because of many factors most athletes are probably not aware of but that the Mucos scientists are, these studies do not apply to other enzyme formulas, and athletes who expect the results reported here in should use the Wobenzym N

How to Use Enzymes for
Prevention and Treatment of Sports Injuries

❖Prefer combination formulas (e.g., Wobenzym N).

❖Prevention is preferred. Athletes should take enzymes prior to physically demanding events.

❖Take enzymes on an empty stomach, at least 45 minutes before a meal, with water or juice.

❖In case of acute injuries, begin taking as soon as possible.
Ingest 5 to 10 tablets three to five times daily when injured.

❖Take a daily maintenance dose of five tablets two to three times daily.

❖If you are already using NSAIDs such as ibuprofen, gradually taper your dose over a several week period; if necessary, consult a health professional.

❖Enzymes are slower acting than drugs such as ibuprofen. For quick relief, use OTC or prescription painkillers for the first few days. But over several days to several weeks, the pain-relieving capabilities of Wobenzym®N will outperform that of the NSAIDs and without toxicity.

Sports Injuries Enzymes Work On...

Acute, traumatic injuries
      Bruises, hematomas, contusions,
      Sprains, Strains, muscle pulls
      Lacerations, abrasions, wounds
      Fractures

Surgical procedures of all kinds

Sciatica and acute lower back pain

Chronic joint conditions
      Rheumatoid arthritis
      Osteoarthritis
      Bursitis
      Tendinitis

formula. For example, injured tissue has a different pH than healthy tissue. Yet, enzymes lose their potency within the body at different levels of pH. The Wobenzym N formula is manufactured to be biochemically active and body ready at pH levels found in both injured and healthy tissues. Many European clinical trials have shown just how effective Wobenzym N can be for anyone suffering inflammation from sports and athletic injuries.

❖ In 1979 Wobenzym N was tested on 45 patients who had sustained sports injuries. Doses ranging from three to ten coated tablets were given. Substantial improvement was seen.[84]

❖ In a second study, similar good results were obtained for 38 of 56 patients with typical sports injuries who responded "very well." Eight other athletes responded "well" with Wobenzym N tablets.[85]

❖ In a double-blind, randomized parallel group study, doctors looked at the effectiveness and tolerance of Wobenzym N in soft-tissue injuries sustained in athletes.[86] The study included 44 patients with various types of injury. Twenty-two patients each took either Wobenzym N or placebo three times daily. The median duration of therapy in both groups was 11 days. The lessening of pain and in the diameter of their hematomas (blood clots) were taken as the primary criteria for statistical evaluation. The results of the study provide impressive evidence that pain and hematomas due to the injury can be reduced significantly and more rapidly with Wobenzym N. The advantage of enzyme therapy is reflected in the reduced need for analgesics and the earlier mobilization in the group taking the preparation. As a result the rate of absence due to injury in this study was substantially shorter.

❖ Perhaps the most physically punishing sport in the world today is boxing. It is with boxers that enzymes have proven to be more than a match for inflammation and pain. In one study, published in *The Practitioner*, systemic oral enzymes were shown to significantly reduce injuries such as cuts, broken vessels, bruising, and sprains when used prior to entering the ring.[87]

❖ So effective are enzymes, in fact, that the American Boxing Association stipulates that athletes should take enzyme preparations a few days before a fight in order to subdue the inflammation caused by trauma, and to accelerate healing.[88, 89]

❖ Similar excellent findings were reported in *The Practitioner* for British soccer players.[90] Among soccer players, enzyme users had fewer missed games and quicker recovery from soft tissue injuries such as bruises and hematomas. Leakage of blood from bruised vessels into body cavities (effusions) was also minimized.

❖ Further good results have been found when enzymes were used for both prevention and for stimulating quicker healing among Germany's Olympic martial arts competitors. Those patients suffering hematomas, swelling, pain, tenderness and impaired mobility experienced much greater improvement in all parameters compared to those athletes not receiving the enzyme mixture.

❖ Finally, when the same enzyme mixture was given to members of the German National Ice Hockey League, it was found that injured players were able to return to competition more rapidly.[91]

❖ Sprained ankles are one of the most common sports injuries. In one placebo–controlled study, 22 of 44 patients with sprained ankles received Wobenzym N for a period of

10 days. Quite apart from markedly reduced swelling and pain, mobility of the injured joint was restored substantially more rapidly in patients taking the enzyme mixture.[92] The duration of disability was shortened significantly. Additional studies validate the great benefits athletes with sprained ankles receive from systemic oral enzymes.[93, 94]

❖ Most recently, Wobenzym N was tested among soccer and karate members of the Ukraine national team. Sixteen of the athletes were given a dose of 10 pills three times daily, starting immediately upon being injured. Fifteen other athletes, in the control group, were treated with compresses, heparin ointment, NSAIDs and various forms of physiotherapy such as electrophoresis with novocaine and hydrocortisone. Size of hematoma, prevalence of edema, severity of pain at rest and on movement duration of suspension of training were among the critical evaluation parameters. Even after two days of treatment with Wobenzym N there was a "noticeable reduction in pain, edema and tension in the affected part of the limb." Without Wobenzym N, this same result required seven to nine days. Athletes in the treated group resumed training 3.5 weeks after starting treatment. Those in the control group required six weeks. No adverse reactions were reported, either. "In view of the very good efficacy of Wobenzym in the treatment of athletes with acute muscle damage, together with the absence of adverse reactions and effects and the fact that it was well tolerated, the extensive use of Wobenzym in sports medicine is recommended."[95]

❖ More than 20 additional studies have further confirmed that enzymes stimulate faster healing and reduced swelling, immobility, inflammation, tenderness, and pain along with improved recovery time.[96]

❖ Tony Cichoke, D.C., a leading sports medicine doctor and enzyme expert, notes that for promoting healing due to sports injuries, "Some feel that enzyme mixtures are superior [to many medically prescribed drugs] because of their comparable efficacy, but minimal side effects."

The Bottom Line

If you're an athlete or simply someone who wants to stay in great shape and enhance their health with daily exercise, supplementing your diet with an enzyme mixture is important for a natural and healthy non-drug approach to chronic inflammation and soreness. Furthermore, enzymes have many other important health benefits, including maintaining healthy blood flow (which may reduce risk of heart disease) and enhancing digestion and immunity.

Enzymes are not as fast acting as typical NSAIDs such as ibuprofen, but over the long run, they are much safer and more effective.

Don't Mask Pain

If you do use pain killers, be sure not to use them before exercising just to get a better work-out. If you mask pain, you'll never know that you are doing damage. Use pain killers afterwards, if you must, only then to help with pain.

Part III

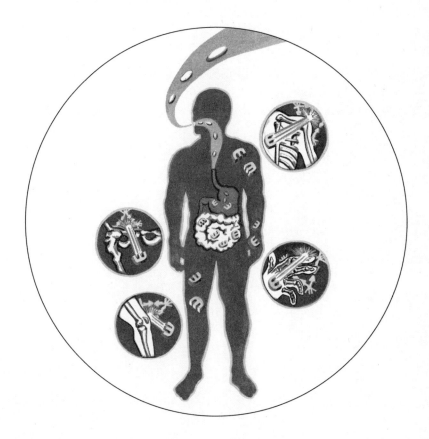

10

Systemic Oral Enzymes and Circulatory Health

So you just heard from your doctor that your cholesterol is out of the world, blood pressure way too high, and that atherosclerosis has turned your heart into a ticking time bomb.

Can we speak heart to heart?

Do you have circulatory problems? Headaches, blood clumping, phlebitis, elevated cholesterol, high blood pressure, angina and other symptoms of poor circulatory or heart health?

Dying of a heart attack or suffering a stroke is no more natural than being run over by an eighteen wheeler. We say that if you die of heart disease, your doctor wasn't doing his job . . . if he or she didn't tell you about systemic oral enzymes.

"With oral enzymes, I can save the life of virtually every one of my heart patients," says noted heart doctor Garry Gordon, M.D., D.O., M.D.(H.).

"For thirty years, I have specialized in keeping people with the most serious and most hopeless heart problems alive," says Dr. Gordon. "In fact, I say if you die of a heart attack or stroke your doctor isn't doing his job because he didn't tell you about systemic oral enzymes. I've treated more than 5,000 patients with heart disease in my nearly thirty years as a heart doctor. I even co-founded an organization dedicated to helping people overcome circulatory and other heart-related problems. That organization is called the American College for Advancement of Medicine (or ACAM for short).

"Our own clinical experience and many clinical studies prove Wobenzym® N can help to dramatically reduce risk of heart attack or stroke and improve your health in other significant ways if you are suffering from thrombosis, heart disorders, phlebitis, edema, varicose veins and other circulatory problems that affect blood flow to and from the brain, lungs, heart, kidneys, liver, and legs.

"As a medical physician who takes on the most hopeless, the most desperate and difficult to heal heart disease patients, I know what kind of miracles Wobenzym N can perform because Wobenzym N is the same formula I have used in my own practice," adds Dr. Gordon. "Now, either my patients are very lucky, or they're doing the right things to stay alive and even reverse their heart disease."

But, we bet your doctor hasn't told you that one of the keys to reversal of heart disease is to reduce the body's overall inflammation levels, boost its immune function, and bolster its ability to fight off bacterial and viral infections.

Inflammation and Heart Disease

A recent report in *The New England Journal of Medicine* said exploration of the relationship between inflammation and heart disease is like "exploring the hidden side of the moon."[97]

"Convincing evidence" has been uncovered that inflammation is strongly linked to heart attacks and stroke, according to Attilio Maseri, M.D., of the Catholic University of the Sacred Heart, Rome, writing in the prestigious medical journal.

A cutting edge nutrition magazine *Nutrition Action Health Letter* highlighted this theory recently in a report, "Inflammation & the Heart."[98, 99]

And a team of scientists from the Harvard Medical School, who have long been involved with the landmark Physicians' Health Study, has also found inflammation leads to heart disease and stroke.

These Harvard University doctors say safe methods of curbing inflammation may be at the "heart" of a sensible cardiovascular health program. Fortunately, Wobenzym N has been proven in clinical trials to safely lower the specific types of inflammation closely linked to heart disease.

These Harvard researchers' findings are literally heartening for the millions of men and women now at risk for heart disease. By curbing excess inflammation, we can literally once again support healthy blood flow throughout our bodies.

The Physicians' Health Study, involving 22,000 male doctors, was halted in 1988 when the researchers discovered that aspirin, a classic anti-inflammatory drug, significantly helped to lower heart disease risk among men. The findings were so significant that the researchers conducting the study believed it was no longer moral or ethical to deny the non-aspirin group this important protective agent.

Doctors Do Not Routinely Test Inflammation Levels

Most doctors today do not know very much about inflammation and heart disease. They do not normally think of inflammation as a cause of heart disease when treating patients, and they rarely measure the body's inflammation levels.

The way to find out the extent to which the body is undergoing significant inflammation is to perform what scientists call a C-reactive protein (CRP) analysis of the blood. When patients have high-normal CRP levels, they should be put on Wobenzym

N to get those levels down because, as the Harvard University study confirms, elevated whole body inflammation is a significant heart attack and stroke risk factor.

In the Physicians' Health Study, Harvard researchers examined levels of C-reactive protein in almost 1,100 men, comparing some 543 who suffered a heart attack with the same number who hadn't.

The doctors found that elevated levels of inflammation throughout the body placed men at a threefold greater risk for heart disease and a twofold increased risk for stroke. The men who benefited most from aspirin had the highest inflammation levels. Yet, dangerous levels of C-reactive protein were found in the high-normal range. This means that what has been long considered a "normal" level of C-reactive protein is actually too high and acceptable levels probably should be revised downward. The problem may be especially severe for anyone already suffering angina.

Aspirin is an anti-inflammatory drug. There is emerging evidence that aspirin reduces risk for colon and breast cancer, and possibly Alzheimer's disease. It is cheap and stable and, for all of its benefits, a potential killer.

Enterically coated or buffered aspirin very possibly are no less irritating to the gastrointestinal tract, claims from manufacturers notwithstanding. There is also a small but very real risk among aspirin users for hemorrhagic stroke. Wobenzym N is as effective as aspirin for reducing inflammation in the body but without any of its terrible side effects.

Can You 'Catch' Heart Disease?

This is where our story takes an unexpected twist . . .

We now know that C-reactive protein is extremely elevated during times of bacterial infection and yet that elevated CRP levels are also linked to higher risk of heart attack and stroke.

Therefore, we must ask the daring, and to some the quite unexpected, question, *Could it be heart disease is not simply a biochemical but also a bacterial malady?*

Could it be that substances such as enzymes, which are so effective at reducing C-reactive protein and heart disease risk, actually do so because they impact the immune system, rev it up, stimulating high levels of bacterial killing chemicals such as interferons?

Angioplasty fails in 60 percent of cases...*but why? Bugs in your pipes! Yes, bacteria.*

Three infectious bacterial agents in particular appear to be related to heart disease; these may also be the criminal culprits that are responsible, in major part, for stimulating high levels of C-reactive protein in the bodies of men and women at risk for heart attack and stroke and, in a sense, for gunking up their arteries, playing a role in plaque build-up that takes us right back to the biological and inflammatory realm of heart disease causation. These three bacterial criminals are cytomegalovirus, *chlamydia pneumoniae*, and *porphyromonas gingivalis.*

"For 17 years, Dr. Joseph Melnick of Houston's Baylor College of Medicine has made a hobby of removing lesions from diseased coronary arteries and testing them for cytomegalovirus (CMV), a common herpes virus," reports the August 11, 1997 *Newsweek*. "It shows up with surprising frequency–and it's looking less harmless all the time. Scientists have long known that CMV can spell trouble for people receiving heart transplants; infected patients are roughly twice as likely as others to lose their new organs, or their lives, to arterial disease."

In 1996, Dr. Stephen Epstein of the National Heart, Lung, and Blood Institute, found that CMV infection increased by four-fold the odds that someone having his arteries reamed out by angioplasty would see them close back up within six months. CMV and heart disease will prove to have an extremely strong link to heart disease, predicts Epstein.

The airborne bacterium *Chlamydia pneumoniae* is known more commonly for causing respiratory illness than the damage it does to the arteries. Yet, surprisingly, a tankerload of recent research has been published linking this bacterium to heart disease.

Over the last year, animal and human studies have pinpointed *Chlamydia pneumoniae* as a possible factor in triggering the inflammatory responses in the tissue lining blood vessels that then leads to plaque obstructions. This bacterium can circulate even inside the body's monocytes, which are large white blood cells that are formed in the bone marrow and spleen and circulate in the blood and tissues as macrophages (which literally translated are the immune system's "big eaters" and are suppose to be the bacterium's worst enemy). In other words, once *Chlamydia pneumoniae* is lodged within our tissues, it becomes an insidious enemy, able to even outsmart our own immune system. Yet beyond causing respiratory distress, Chlamydia, we now know, contributes to the buildup of arterial plaque.

British researchers have found that having high antibodies to *Chlamydia pneumoniae* predispose people to a second heart attack. The patients of Dr. Sandeep Gupta, of St. George's Hospital, London, with evidence of the bacteria were as much as four times more likely than other patients to suffer further heart problems over an 18-month period that they were studied. The British researcher has found that antibiotic treatments reduce the risk of heart attack. A three-day course of the antibiotic azithromycin seems to work, according to Dr. Gupta. But antibiotics are a quick fix. Besides, what bacteria are not killed may reproduce and populate the body with additional antibiotic-resistant strains.

Enzymes also work, but they're systemic and actually rev up the immune system, enabling the body to do its own business, to take care of its own internal affairs without requiring the shotgun approach of antibiotic therapy.

Floss or die!

Do you floss your teeth as often as you should? You might want to be sure you do–especially after learning about this third troublemaker, *Porphyomonas gingivitis.*

Responsible also for gum disease, this bacterium is now also known for its damaging effects on the linings of the arteries.

According to the work of Dr. Raul Garcia of the Boston VA Outpatient Clinic and part of the VA Normative Aging Study, over a 25–year period some 1,100 men were studied. They were healthy at the start, but the men with the worst gums had twice the heart–attack rate of their peers with healthy gums and odorless breath. Their stroke rate was three times as high. The bacterium has also been found at the scene of the crime: in diseased carotid arteries. Again, this leads us to suspect this bacterium may also cause heart disease. Wobenzym N can help by doing more than simply quelling the inflammatory symptoms associated with the body's infectious state. It enhances healing by favorably modulating the body's immune system so that the body actually vanquishes this and other harmful strains of bacteria.

How Wobenzym N Destroys Heart Disease-Causing Bacteria

Wobenzym N directly impacts human immune function by stimulating the following immune enhancing events in the human body:

❖ *Induction of optimal amounts of tumor necrosis factor and inter-leukins.* This systemic enzyme formula leads to a dose-dependent increased formation of tumor necrosis factor (TNF–a), interleukin 1–b and interleukin 6. These tough cops kill dangerous cells and tissues circulating in the body, as well as mount attacks on bacteria and viruses.

❖ *Macrophage and killer activation.* The activity of bacteria–con-suming macrophages is increased up to 700 percent within only 10 minutes following Wobenzym N enzyme treatments in the test tube in German studies. The activity of natural killer cells went up 1,300 percent during the same time.[101]

❖ *Selective Destruction of Infectious Agents.* The proteolytic enzymes added to cell cultures cause loss of nuclei, sub-stantial disintegration and, finally, complete destruction of cancer cells, while leaving healthy cells unaffected. This cancer cell necrosis typically spreads continuously from a single point of origin until the margins of healthy tissue have been reached.[102, 103, 104]

In another study, Wobenzym N was studied for its ability to reduce C–reactive protein levels after operative dentistry in a randomized, placebo–controlled, double–blind study.[106] Prior to surgical dental intervention, 36 patients were prescribed ten tablets of Wobenzym twice daily. In the control group, 44 patients received placebo. This dosage was continued until the seventh postoperative day. None of the test subjects received any preoperative therapy with other anti–inflammatory drugs. By day three, C–reactive protein levels were threefold lower in the group taking Wobenzym N compared to patients in the control group.

In the most recent study, 35 patients were treated by Dr. I.K. Sledsewskaja and other doctors at the Ukraine Scientific Institute of Cardiology, Kiev. These patients were given Wobenzym N following heart attack and received 9 coated tablets daily total in three divided doses of three tablets three times daily.

According to Dr. Sledsewskaja the immune system goes through pronounced changes following a heart attack. Therefore, he reasoned, Wobenzym N may be beneficial to administer following myocardial infarct (MI).

After treatment with Wobenzym, patients experienced "a significant drop in total cholesterol and LDL (low density lipoproteins), a trend toward a lower triglyceride concentration and reduction in atherogenesis," says Dr. Sledsewskaja.[107]

The doctor concluded, "Our preliminary results prove that we are fully justified in administering Wobenzym N to patients after MI as a preparation that corrects the immune status and lowers lipid concentrations." In a personal interview, Dr. Sledsewskaja adds that preliminary data indicates that Wobenzym is able to markedly lower overall inflammation and C-reactive protein levels after a heart attack as well.

Today, we finally have a safe tool for reducing levels of C-reactive protein in the body and therefore risk of heart attack or stroke.

In fact, enzymes support healthy immune function and can help with a host of other maladies.

Many European doctors believe that enzymes are a safe, natural tool for achieving the anti-inflammatory effects derived from aspirin but without aspirin's complications.

Wobenzym N is good medicine.

Health Professionals Comment on the Use of Wobenzym N for Heart and Circulatory Health

"'Doctor, can you heal me? I don't want heart disease to cut my life short. I've got so much to live for!' I hear this often desperate

---

Smart Advice for Medical Consumers

If your doctor has you on aspirin or other blood thinners and you wish to use systemic oral enzymes, this medical decision should be made in consultation with your health professional.

"I have found as a heart doctor that enzymes help to favorably influence circulatory disorders and can reduce my patients' need for aspirin," says Dr. Gordon. "I especially recommend enzymes to my patients who are not on aspirin but wish to reduce their risk of a heart attack or stroke.

Systemic oral enzymes can be used alone or in conjunction with other oral chelators such as *Ginkgo biloba*, garlic, and oral or intravenous EDTA, all of which have the ability to beneficially alter blood coagulation.

---

plea from new patients almost daily. Heart disease is our nation's number one killer. Half of all Americans who die this year will die from it," says Dr. Gary Wikholm, M.D., a board-certified specialist in family medicine and also a specialist in emergency medicine and obstetrics, a qualified medical evaluator in occupational medicine for the state of California and clinical instructor in the Family Medicine Glendale-Adventist Family Practice Residency Program, which is part of Loma Linda University. He is also a clinical instructor in emergency medicine for the Ventura County Medical Center. "Look," he says, "in the emergency room, I see the victims. Unfortunately, I can't always help them because for 400,000, people a year, their very first symptom is their last— a fatal heart attack. You can significantly reduce your risk for heart disease and stroke, and Wobenzym N is a powerful tool for doing so. Except for a few rare types of heart malfunctions, *you can take control of your heart's health and heal yourself without dangerous drugs and surgery! And systemic oral enzymes are a key tool for my patients, especially those who prefer natural healing pathways to reduce inflammation without aspirin's potential complications."*

"Wobenzym N is a medically validated pathway for naturally reducing the body's inflammatory levels and thereby reducing the risk of heart and circulatory disorders," says Megan Shields, M.D. "I urge my patients to take full advantage of natural healing pathways. Wobenzym N is thoroughly documented in prestigious journals to address underlying inflammatory conditions which can contribute to risk for heart disease and stroke. What's more, because it is completely nontoxic, I know it is safe for my patients to use long-term. For many patients, I would recommend it over aspirin."

"Often overlooked in the heart equation are women. Women are more likely than men to die from a heart attack, receive inferior treatment, and may even go for years without their heart disease being diagnosed," says Dr. Shields. "That's why I believe women will benefit greatly from using systemic oral enzymes daily. I strongly recommend Wobenzym N to many of my women patients."

How to Use Enzymes for Circulatory Health

Take three to five tablets two to three times daily on an empty stomach 30 to 45 minutes before meals with water or juice.

If you are using NSAIDs such as aspirin for heart disease prevention but are suffering complications from their use or you are using other blood thinners, work with your doctor to gradually.

11

Enhancing the Healing Response with Systemic Oral Enzymes

In the treatment of many acute and chronic inflammatory conditions, doctors recommend use of a combination of prescription and over the counter drugs. In cases of bronchitis, for example, drugs that stimulate secretory activities (i.e., secretolytics), antibiotics and NSAIDs may all be recommended. Many times these drugs are absolutely necessary.

What is most amazing about systemic oral enzymes is that they clearly enhance the benefits to be derived from the drugs doctors recommend. Sometimes they may even make it so that persons suffering from the acute inflammatory and related conditions detailed in this chapter do not even require drugs–and, at the very least, can reduce the dosage required, thereby making the use of medical drugs safer; in other words, systemic oral enzymes can enhance the efficacy of such drugs. In other cases, Wobenzym N has been proven to reduce the need for chronic use of drugs, including antibiotics, by making sure they work right the first time. It is really quite amazing. Again, we have enormous clinical validation, which makes this application of systemic oral enzymes very exciting for both practitioners and their patients. Let's look at some of the conditions for which systemic oral enzymes are particularly beneficial.

Acute and Chronic Bronchitis

There are different types of bronchitis, an inflammation of the upper respiratory pathway involving the bronchial tubes and lungs.

Acute bronchitis is an illness which is increasing in incidence. The tracheal and bronchial system are often involved in the common cold and in infections with adenoviruses, mycoviruses, echoviruses and rhinoviruses as well as in other infectious diseases including measles, influenza, whooping cough, and typhoid fever.

Very often, bacterial secondary infections resulting from germs such as staphylococci, streptococci, and haemophilus influenza do not occur until the primary immune response is underway. In this case, viruses weaken the entire defense system, making the body susceptible to these secondary bacterial infections.

Acute bronchitis can also be promoted by chronic or acute exposition to such irritants as dust, smoking, environmental poisons, highly toxic aerosols and gases.

There is also chronic bronchitis. The World Health Organization defines chronic bronchitis as a persistent inflammation of the tracheobronchial tree which is associated with productive cough for at least two to three months in two successive years. Obstruction of the respiratory tract may occur, depending on the intensity of immune response. Should this process become chronic, pulmonary emphysema often develops as a further sequel or an accompanying illness. Approximately 20% of the adult male population in the industrialized nations has chronic bronchitis. However, only a small proportion of these individuals suffer substantial physical impairment. Respiratory obstruction and emphysema increase appreciably after the fifth decade of life. Male smokers are affected more severely than women who smoke.

Smoking, nitrous gases sulfur dioxide in the air and other inhaled irritants promote respiratory tract infections and chronic inflammations by irritating the mucous membranes; edema of the bronchial wall and chronic infiltration by inflammatory cells may also occur.

Therapeutically, it is essential to eliminate the noxae. Incipient bacterial superinfection must be treated with antibiotics. Bronchodilatory agents, secretolytic drugs and, tentatively, even corticosteroids, in addition to physiotherapy, are standard procedures to achieve drainage.

Enzymes lead to a reduction of the mucosal swelling and facilitate the removal of lymph. They serve as a "vehicle" for antibiotics and increase their local concentration in the respiratory tissues. Enzymes degrade and eliminate inflammatory products and antigen-antibody complexes, improve the supply of oxygen by reducing the blood viscosity and break down microthrombi and fibrin depositions. In stubborn cases of bronchitis, phlegm is loosened, which is generally noticed as temporarily increased expectoration.[108]

How to Use Wobenzym N for Bronchitis . . .

The dosage should not be less than three coated tablets of Wobenzym N three times daily.

Be sure to use Wobenzym N with your antibiotics. The combination of antibiotics and enzymes together with the usual therapeutic procedures leads to astonishingly rapid improvements and a good therapeutic outcome.

Dr. Grimminger confirmed that all exudative inflammatory lung conditions can be influenced positively by enzyme mixtures.

Dr. A. Grimminger was interested in the enzyme treatment of pulmonary, bronchial and pleural diseases as early as 1953. He has administered Wobenzym N since 1968 and, on the basis of his case studies, subsequently evaluated the efficacy of oral enzymes for diseases of the respiratory organs.[109] According to Dr. Grimminger, oral enzymes lead to reduced swelling of the bronchial mucosa as well as to liquefaction of the secretion and, consequently, to improved expectoration and ventilation in cases of both acute and chronic bronchitis.

In October 2005, a research team from Tbilisi State Medical University, Georgia, studied Wobenzym N in children with recurrent obstructive bronchitis. A total of 27 patients with recurrent obstructive bronchitis (at least 3 episodes of obstructive bronchitis per year) of 5–15 years of age were studied. Wobenzym N was administered for three months. Analysis of the data, obtained after treatment, demonstrated decrease of the Daily Symptom Score and an increase of Symptom Free Days, as well as an improvement in spirometric indices. "According to these data, it was concluded, that systemic enzyme preparation Wobenzym N should be used as a supporting measure in combination treatment of recurrent obstructive bronchitis."

Under appropriate antibiotic treatment selected by resistance testing, clearing of the bronchial system occurs rapidly, expectoration is reduced, cough is alleviated and secretion is transformed to a seromucous, whitish fluid.

Sinusitis

Bronchitis is often found concomitantly with chronic sinusitis. Sinusitis usually develops by continuous spreading of rhinitis, but may also arise following injury.

Increasing exposure to environmental pollutants as well as the ever more frequent prevalence of congenital immune deficiency is thought to be responsible for the growing incidence of chronic inflammations of the nasal sinuses.

Chronic sinusitis is difficult to treat. Today, operative therapy with currettage of the mucosa is often considered inadequate, as it is generally limited to correction of the airway blockage. Medical therapy includes the prescription of secretolytics and locally applied decongestants. Furthermore, a number of antibiotics are available, although they rarely attain effective concentrations in the mucosa or bone of the nasal sinuses.

Healing of the chronic inflammation is seldom possible with the usual conservative measures. Surgical irritation with instillation of antibiotics and corticosteroids entails the risk of sensitization of the mucous membranes. Corticosteroids additionally interfere with the defensive mechanisms which are already somewhat impaired.

The goal of oral enzymes is to support the normal inflammatory process and the natural clearance functions while stimulating the immune system. With this in mind, oral enzymes have been applied successfully by many therapists. As early as 1967, Dr. R.E. Ryan examined the therapeutic effect of bromelain on acute sinusitis in a double-blind study.[110]

The efficacy of Wobenzym N in acute sinusitis was verified by Dr. R. Wohlrab in a randomized, double-blind, parallel group clinical study. Forty patients with roentgenologically and sonographically verified acute sinusitis (maxillary, frontal or ethmoidal sinusitis) took part in this study. Twenty patients each were assigned to the enzyme and the diclofenac groups. Both groups were matched with respect to age, sex, height, weight, swelling of the middle meatus of the nose, pus, ultrasonic findings, fever, headache, toothache in the upper jaw and sensation of pressure.

The enzyme received one measuring spoon of granulated Wobenzym N twice daily and two capsules of placebo, whereas the diclofenac group received one measuring spoon of granulated placebo twice daily and two capsules of diclofenac. Improvement of headache and toothache as well as in the sensation of pressure were taken as major criteria for statistical evaluation.

None of the criteria examined revealed a significant difference between the two groups after 14 days of therapy. Wobenzym therapy therefore was equivalent to treatment with diclofenac.[111]

Prostatitis

The prostate gland and seminal vesicle (the male appendages) form a unit embryologically, anatomically and functionally. The prostate, an organ which is well supplied with blood and normally undergoes periods of congestion, is the central point of this organ system, and is liable to be afflicted with acute or chronic infections. Approximately 30% of males between the age of 25 and 40 years with prostate complaints have true prostatitis and 30% a genitoanal syndrome, the remainder having other pathological prostatic conditions. Because of the similarity of symptoms, it is difficult even for experts to differentiate the various clinical syndromes. Aside from the typical complex of complaints, acute prostatitis is often accompanied by fever and chills. In addition to analgesics, therapy includes high-dosed chemotherapy with antibiotics. Should the inflammation not be brought under control, a prostatic abscess or other condition may develop. In spite of specific chemotherapy, acute prostatitis regardless of the causative agent may develop into a chronic inflammation.

Table 11.1

Effects of Simultaneously Administered Hydrolytic Enzymes on Antibiotic Serum Levels

Chemical preparation	Preparation (μg/ml)	Preparation + Wobenzym° N (μg/ml)	Increase in %
Minocycline	0.6	0.7	17
Cephradine	1.1	1.2	9
Doxycyline	0.5	0.7	40
Cefadroxil	2.4	2.6	8
Amoxicillin	1.2	1.5	25
Tetroxoprim	24.0	38.0	17
Trimethoprim	1.4	1.7	21
Tetracycline	0.9	1.1	22
Ampicillin	0.4	0.5	25
Sulfadiazine	36.0	39.0	8

Serum levels of antibiotics 8 hours after administration

Oral Enzymes in Prostatitis

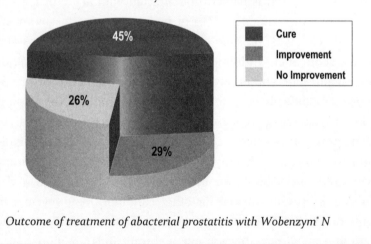

Outcome of treatment of abacterial prostatitis with Wobenzym° N

Chronic prostatitis, on the other hand, proceeds blandly and without fever. It is often the residual condition following acute prostatitis, although it may also ascend along the ducts or spread via the blood. A target-specific chemotherapy can only be carried out if it is possible to verify bacteria. As in other pathological prostatic conditions, treatment is limited to herbal sedatives and agents for stimulating blood flow, regulation of the bowels, sitz baths and mild hydrotherapy.

Drs. S. Barsom, K. Sasse-Rollenhagen and A. Bettermann concentrated their interest on bacterial prostatitis. In a randomized, double-blind study on 44 patients, they administered Wobenzym N together with antibiotics to treat the acute inflammation.[112]

Twenty-two patients of the group receiving the actual preparation were given five coated Wobenzym N tablets three times daily over a period of ten days in a combined regimen. An improvement in complaints occurred earlier and lasted longer for these patients, and, in comparison to the 22 patients of the placebo group, the measures of serum levels of the administered chemotherapeutics were substantially higher (see Table 11.1).

Dr. Barsom considers Wobenzym N a substantial enrichment of the therapeutic options for successfully treating inflammatory disease.

In contrast to Barsom, Dr. E.W. Ruggendorff and co-investigators examined the efficacy of Wobenzym N in a prospective study on 60 patients with abacterial prostatitis. The patients received five coated tablets of Wobenzym N three times daily as a single agent therapy for six weeks. Subjective and objective complaints or findings were determined before beginning therapy. A sensation of tension or pressure in the perineal region, inguinal pain and pain radiating into the testicles as well as disorders of sexual function were considered subjective complaints, whereas white blood cells in the urine, palpatory findings in the rectum, the immunological examination of the ejaculate, uroflowmetric data and the results of roentgenological examinations were regarded as objective criteria.

Data of 49 patients without complicating factors could be evaluated. The outcome of treatment of abacterial prostatitis with Wobenzym N was that 45% of patients were cured and 29% experienced marked improvement.[113]

Cystitis and Lower Urinary Tract Infections (UTIs)

Despite ever improving antibiotic therapy, 10% of the population is affected by infections of the urinary tract, most often afflicting the bladder as well. Acute primary or secondary cystitis usually involves an infectious inflammation of the bladder mucosa. As in all urinary tract infections, the characteristic quartet of bacterial pathogens which appear again and again is also encountered here: *E. coli, Enterococci, Proteus bacteria* and *Staphylococcus aureus*, in a mono or polyinfection. Cystitis can develop by extension from the kidneys or ascend via the urethra, spreading systemically. Due to their short urethra, women are more liable to be afflicted with ascending infections. Contributory factors are cold, urinary retention and changes in the local environment due to hormonal factors as well as prior damage by allergic cystitis, radiation cystitis or toxic cystitis (effects of chemical substances).

In addition to measures as bed rest, fluid intake and analgesics, the causative agents respond to specific chemotherapy.

Cystitis and UTIs tend to become chronic, especially if the mucosa was damaged previously. Chronic cystitis and UTIs often proceed intermittently. The deeper layers of the bladder wall are usually also involved in the inflammatory process.

Enzymes interrupt the causative pathogenic sequence of chronic inflammation. They cause dissipation of inflammatory edema and counteract the pathogenicity of inflammatory products and antigen–antibody complexes by causing their breakdown and elimination. Aside from relieving pain, enzymes stimulate the microcirculation and inhibit the further development and chronification of the process.[114, 115]

Encouraged by the success of their therapy on prostatitis, Dr. S. Barsom and co–investigators performed further clinical examinations with Wobenzym N on patients with cystitis and UTIs. They treated 56 patients with a combination of Wobenzym N and antibiotics. Twenty–eight of the test subjects each suffered from either cystitis or UTI. Laboratory chemical, urinalysis and the bacteriological examination served as investigation parameters.

Wobenzym N increased the serum concentration of all antibiotics and chemotherapeutic drugs given.

Overall, Dr. Barsom sees Wobenzym N as an ideal partner for specific chemotherapy against an infective agent. A complete cure without recurrence was achieved only by this combination therapy.[116]

Pelvic Inflammatory Disease

Pelvic inflammatory disease (PID) primarily afflicts women of child–bearing age. It is a classical example of the beneficial effects of Wobenzym N on a chronic, recurrent disease. Prevention of pelvic congestion and the subsequent impairment of physical activity or possible infertility are the major considerations of treatment. Acute and subacute PID requires antibiotic therapy in all cases. Anti–inflammatory therapy is frequently prescribed– including occasionally use of corticosteroids. Nevertheless, the

Table 11.2

Oral Enzymes in Pelvic Inflammatory Disease

Evaluation of success	Wobenzym'N	Standard therapy
Improved	0	13 = 26.5%
Chronic	–	8
Subacute	–	2
Acute	–	3
Substantially improved	22 = 43.1%	33 = 67.4%
Chronic	2	15
Subacute	6	11
Acute	14	7
Without complaints	29 = 56.9%	3 = 6.1%
Chronic	9	1
Subacute	9	2
Acute	11	–
Total	51	49

Results of therapy with the Wobenzym N preparation as compared to control groups

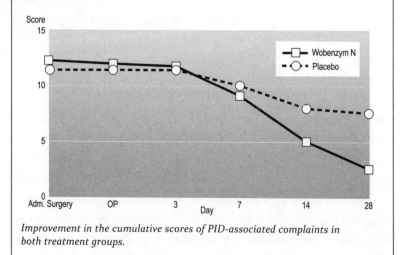

Improvement in the cumulative scores of PID-associated complaints in both treatment groups.

long-term use of NSAIDs may also result in adverse effects which, in spite of therapeutic success, are not justified.

Dr. F.-W. Dittmar first used Mucos systemic oral enzymes (Wobenzym N) in his practice with PID patients and observed good outcomes. This led to his randomized, double-blind study on 100 patients with PID.[117] The group given the enzyme preparation received five coated tablets of Wobenzym N three times daily whereas the control group received a NSAID drug in the usual dosage. Dr. Dittmar additionally prescribed an antibiotic for patients with subacute or acute PID. The average time of treatment was 16 or 17 days.

Dr. Dittmar performed examinations at the start of therapy and on the seventh and fourteenth days, including palpation, white blood counts, erythrocyte sedimentation rate, bacteriological examination and pelviscopy. Wobenzym N therapy led to an improvement in laboratory data and palpatory gynecological findings within a short time. Most of the patients using Wobenzym N were already free of complaints after only 14 days of therapy. In fact, as you can see from Table 11.2, nearly 57% of patients using Wobenzym N were without complaints after therapy, whereas only about six percent using the NSAIDs were without complaints. In total, 100% of patients reported their condition as "substantially improved" or were "without complaints" compared to only 73.5% of patients using NSAIDs.

Herpes Zoster (Shingles)

A particularly virulent member of the herpes virus family, the varicella–zoster virus causes shingles, a condition in which severe burning of the area often precedes the occurrence of blisters. The blisters most often afflict the side of the trunk but can also attack

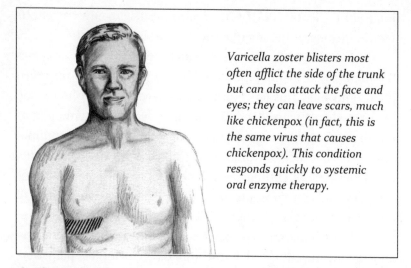

Varicella zoster blisters most often afflict the side of the trunk but can also attack the face and eyes; they can leave scars, much like chickenpox (in fact, this is the same virus that causes chickenpox). This condition responds quickly to systemic oral enzyme therapy.

the face and eyes–they can leave scars, much like chickenpox (in fact, this is the same virus that causes chickenpox).

In 1964, German doctors began using enzyme combinations for the treatment of patients with herpes zoster. The results were astounding; pain was reduced within three days with accelerated healing. A study comparing the effects of enzyme therapy with acyclovir (Zovirax) has shown there are no significant differences in the effects on pain or the healing of skin eruptions. Postherpetic neuralgic appeared substantially later under systemic enzyme therapy.[118] Many of the systemic oral enzyme studies done today were performed using Wobenzym N or other closely related formulas manufactured by the German enzyme company, Mucos Pharma GmbH.

How to Use Wobenzym N for Herpes Zoster (Shingles)

Take five tablets three times daily (on an empty stomach) at least 35 to 45 minutes before meals or not less than 45 minutes after meals.

Lysine Can Help

Lysine, an amino acid, is often beneficial in helping to prevent recurrences of some types of herpes outbreaks.[119, 120] That is because the herpes virus requires another amino acid, arginine, to reproduce. As lysine closely resembles arginine, sometimes the herpes virus mistakes the former for the latter, thus inhibiting its replication.[121] Foods high in arginine include chocolate, peanuts, almonds, nuts and seeds. Foods rich in lysine include vegetables, beans, fish, turkey and chicken. Take 500 to 1,000 mg of lysine with every meal. Lysine can be purchased from your local health food store.

Keep in mind that lysine alone will not control herpes, and that each of these natural medicines may be used in combination or to augment other anti-viral medications prescribed by your doctor.

Ulcerative Colitis and Crohn's Disease

Ulcerative colitis is recognized as a chronically recurrent inflammation of the large intestine. Crohn's disease is a chronic inflammatory disease which begins with the formation of granulomas and can be found throughout the entire intestinal tract, although it is most frequently seen in the ileum and colon.

Both conditions may be accompanied by conjunctivitis and other inflammatory conditions throughout the body.

Although corticosteroids and sulfa drugs are sometimes used, no satisfactory therapy is yet known.

Therapeutic success with Wobenzym N has been reported in numerous case histories. Dr. C. Neuhofer reports of a 32-year-old female patient who repeatedly suffered from severe episodes of ulcerative colitis with some 20 stools a day–a classic picture of an ulcerative, intestinal inflammation confirmed with colonoscopy.

Corticosteroid and sulfasalzine therapy were poorly tolerated. The patient also demonstrated extensive anemia.

Dr. Neuhofer began therapy with 30 coated tablets of Wobenzym N given in small dosages throughout the day together with vitamins. After only one week, the number of stools per day had been reduced to six and laboratory values had returned to normal.

How to Use Wobenzym N for Ulcerative Colitis and Crohn's Disease

After therapeutic success with up to 30 Wobenzym N tablets daily in small divided doses becomes evident, long-term follow-up treatment should be continued with three to five coated tablets of Wobenzym N three times daily for ulcerative colitis and Crohn's disease.

Ulcerative colitis that has persisted for a number of years promotes the development of cancer. Today, it is thought that Crohn's disease has also demonstrated increased risk of cancer. For this reason, it is advisable to continue with Wobenzym N therapy indefinitely as a cancer preventive.

Pancreatitis

Pancreatitis is a rapidly progressive disease. Inflammation of the pancreas may eventually lead to tissue death. The acute form is frequently found in connection with alcohol-related disease, biliary disease and as a postoperative complication following surgical interventions in the abdominal cavity. High cholesterol, hyperthyroidism, gastric ulcers, mumps and use of corticosteroids may also contribute to the onset of this disease. In about 20% of cases, the cause may be an immune malfunction.

Analgesics are almost always necessary. Mortality ranges from 20% to 80%.

In contrast to acute pancreatitis, the chronic form is often free of pain. It is generally accompanied by weight loss, fatty food intolerance, meteorism, and signs of diabetes.

Wobenzym N may offer important help. In one study, Moser treated more than 70 patients who suffered from pancreatitis. Initial results appear to be promising.

Dr. R. Chappa–Alvarez has been using Wobenzym N at the Hospital Civil in Guadalajara, Mexico, since 1981 and is currently conducting a controlled clinical study on 40 patients with verified pancreatitis.[122] Preliminary data from this study show that Wobenzym N promotes improvement in the clinical picture of inflammation of the pancreas, reduces the pain and lethality of rapidly progressive pancreatitis, decreases the rate of inflammatory reactions, assists in avoiding complications and shortens the duration of hospitalization. In the group receiving the oral enzyme therapy, a distinct improvement in abdominal pain was already seen beginning on the second day of therapy. The average hospital stay in the enzyme preparation group of 9.3 days was substantially shorter than that in the control group (14.2 days). In the preparation group, 80% of the patients could be discharged within the first 11 days. In contrast, this was only possible for 55% of the patients in the control group. In summary, these preliminary results show that patients with acute pancreatitis treated with Wobenzym N demonstrate astonishing improvements in clinical symptoms and a reduction in the rate of complications. In particular, patients with numerous accompanying conditions, including kidney disease and diabetes, responded well to Wobenzym N.

Therapy must be continued to prevent renewed symptoms of pain and elevated temperatures.

Enzymes Help Eradicate
Most Common STD: Chlamydia

Chlamydiae are a type of microscopic organism that are not bacteria, viruses, or fungi. Chlamydiae cause one of the most common sexually transmitted diseases (STDs), nongonococcal urethritis, a urinary tract inflammation whose symptoms in both sexes include pain when urinating and a watery, mucous discharge. This STD may result in pelvic inflammatory disease and cause inflammation and infection of the uterus, fallopian tubes, ovaries and surrounding tissues, causing infertility even in asymptomatic carriers.

At the present time, chlamydial infections are one of the most common causes of inflammation in the genitourinary system in both men and women. Although antibiotics are effective, there are no optimal methods for managing these infections.

The recommended regimens provide clinical results, but, still, in 30 to 50 percent of cases there is no etiological cure (elimination of the causative agent). The use of conventional antibacterial drugs frequently only transforms an infection into a latent chronic form and increases the likelihood of selection of drug-resistant strains. However, systemic oral enzymes may be just the answer people with this STD have been seeking–at least according to the latest research presented in 1996 at the Second Russian Symposium on Oral Enzyme Therapy, held in St. Petersburg, Russia.

Systemic Enzymes Enhance Antibiotics

Recently, a clinical trial was undertaken to study the effect of Wobenzym® N and its ability to wipe-out any traces of this virulent microorganism. The researchers also examined this preparation's effect on the interferon system in patients with inflammatory diseases of the genital tract.

The study participants consisted of 68 women and 91 men attending the Scientific Center for Obstetrics, Gynecology and Perinatology of the Russian Academy of Medical Science because of inflammatory diseases of the genitourinary system and/or infertility.[123]

Some 93 percent of the women were suffering vaginal discharge and pain in the lower part of the abdomen; 77 percent joint pain; 91 percent itching (pruritus); 72 percent difficult or painful urination (dysuria); 28 percent inflammation of the cervix (cervicitis); and 41 percent inflammation of the mucous membrane that covers the exposed portion of the eyeball and lines the inner surface of the eyelids (i.e., conjunctivitis, a symptom of a form of the chlaymidial-related disease called trachoma). Some 57 percent of the women had been diagnosed with infertility of unknown cause and 35 percent had suffered chronic miscarriages. They were in dire need of help in ridding themselves of their infectious state.

The main disorders in the men were pruritus, urethral pain, abnormally large amounts of blood in portions of the body (hyperemia); minor urethral discharges; and pain in the perineum, anus and lumbar areas.

In some cases there were sexual problems such as erectile dysfunction and reduced duration of intromission. Although 83.5 percent of men did not report problems with the genitourinary system, nevertheless, a reduction in quality of ejaculate was observed in the majority of men (about 80.9 percent) in the form of various combinations of low sperm counts (oligospermia); weak sperm (asthenospermia); deformed sperm (teratozoospermia) and pus mixed with sperm (pyospermia); with a predominance of asthenozoospermia.

In the first group, 29 women and 20 men received two 10-day courses one week apart of conventional antibiotics.

In the second group 25 women and 37 men were given the same treatment with intramuscular injection of one bottle a day of chymotrypsin.

In the third group, 14 women and 34 men received antibiotics and oral Wobenzym N at a dose of 5 tablets three times a day.

The conventional course of antibiotics produced clinical recovery only in 17.2 percent of the women with chlamydial infections. Indeed, chlamydia remained in the smears of 72.4 percent of patients after treatment.

The antibiotic treatment was greatly increased if proteolytic enzymes were used, either intramuscularly or orally, in combination with antibiotics. The injected enzymes however were both physically painful and produced allergic reactions.

For practical purposes, it is the orally administered formula with which typical medical consumers should be concerned. In the case of Wobenzym N, its use resulted in 62.5 percent to 66.7 percent of women showing complete clinical recovery with clean smears. All women experienced good results.

The therapeutic effect of Wobenzym N in the treatment of male genitourinary inflammatory diseases also enhanced antibiotic treatment. Complete recovery was obtained far more frequently with additional use of orally administered enzymes.

In fact, 89.5 percent of men experienced complete elimination of the causative agent.

How Enzymes Help Recovery from Chlamydia

The mode of action in using Wobenzym N seems to be a change in interferon status. Interferons are proteins produced by virus-infected cells. They inhibit reproduction of invading viruses and induce resistance to further infection. Systemic oral enzyme therapy appears to normalize serum interferon concentrations.

Before treatment, most patients with chronic infections had a reduced capacity for production of both white blood cells and interferons. In 58 percent of patients taking Wobenzym N the capacity of lymphocytes for synthesis of interferons was restored with in 24 hours. Two days after starting treatment with Wobenzym N, lymphocyte capacity to produce interferons was restored in 73 percent of patients. None of the patients taking oral enzymes experienced any allergic or adverse reactions.

The study shows systemic oral enzymes given in multidrug therapy with antibiotics greatly increased efficacy against inflammatory disease of the genital tract caused by chlamydial infections. Recovery is accompanied not only by an improvement in clinical situation, but also by more effective elimination of causative agent.

In October 2006, researchers reported in the October Russian language publication of Georgia Medical News found that enzyme–immunomodification therapy in women with urogenital chlamydiosis could be very help. "The most expressive clinical effect was received using the combination of the antibiotic, enzymes and immuno–correction."

In October 2006, researchers reported in the October Russian language publication of Georgia Medical News found that enzyme–immunomodification therapy in women with urogenital chlamydiosis could be very help. "The most expressive clinical effect was received using the combination of the antibiotic, enzymes and immuno–correction."

What to Do . . .

If you or a loved one suffer from chlamydia, it is important to consult with your health professional. If your health professional prescribes antibiotics, be sure to also take five Wobenzym N tablets three times daily 30 to 45 minutes before meals.

12

On the Horizon: New Healing Miracles with Systemic Oral Enzymes

The innovative scientists affiliated with the parent company of Wobenzym N, Mucos Pharma GmbH, continue to research new and exciting applications for systemic oral enzymes. We want to tell you about the cutting-edge research now occurring in several of these fields.

Juvenile Diabetes

One of the great health tragedies of childhood is juvenile diabetes. In such cases, the child's immune system B cells (for not yet well understood reasons) produce protein molecules (antibodies) that attack the body's own tissues, in this case insulin producing cells in the pancreas (islets of Langerhans). Now that these antibodies have been clearly identified by medical scientists, it is known that fifty percent of such children with these antibodies will develop what we typically call Type I juvenile diabetes.

There is now genuine hope on the horizon that no child should ever have to fall prey to this disease. Because juvenile diabetes is a disease in which the immune system attacks its own host, it is thought to be an auto-immune disease. For this reason, scientists believe systemic oral enzymes, which have proven helpful with other auto-immune diseases, may find another important medical application and help to *prevent* juvenile diabetes.

In experimental studies, an enzyme mixture (Phlogenzym® from Mucos Pharma GmbH–very similar to Wobenzym N) inhibited the occurrence of this disease; these important findings have convinced health experts in Germany that systemic oral enzymes could have the same preventive impact on diabetes-prone children.

Can enzymes benefit children at risk for diabetes? The experimental evidence is promising; we don't know yet for sure.

Systemic Oral Enzymes: Significant New Help for Multiple Sclerosis

Multiple sclerosis (MS) is yet another tragic disease that strikes relatively young persons and has no known cure. Systemic oral enzymes, however, offer real hope.

More than 100,000 individuals in Germany and worldwide many more than one million individuals suffer from MS. The disease is seen much more frequently in cold, damp climactic region than in the warmer countries. Independent of these climactic zones, however, specific population groups are afflicted more frequently with this disease. MS occurs about twice as frequently among women as in men. It usually begins between the ages of 15 and 40.

In fact, MS is the third most cause of severe disability in patients in the United States between the ages of 15 and 50, reports Reuven Sandyk, M.D., M.Sc. in the *Journal of Alternative and Complementary Medicine.*

"The cause of the disease and its pathogenesis remain unknown," reports Sandyk. "The last 20 years have seen only meager advances in the development of effective treatments for the disease. No specific treatment modality can cure the disease or alter its long-term course and eventual outcome."

Current Treatment

Corticosteroids are a mainstay of therapy for MS with their main benefit being accelerating recovery from exacerbation of the condition. Severe exacerbations are often treated with intravenous methylprednisolone. Beta-interferon, an immunomodulator, has been recently approved by the Food and Drug Administration for patients with relapsing-remitting MS who are ambulatory. Interferon reduces the frequency, severity, and duration of exacerbations, but its impact on preventing disability over the long-term is not established. Copolymer-1 is a synthetic protein comprised of the major amino acids in myelin basic protein. It is given by injection daily to induce suppression of the immune response against myelin and to promote immune tolerance. Recent trials suggest that copolymer-1 treatment results in a mild amelioration of acute MS episodes, but mainly in patients with very early MS. Patients with primary or secondarily progressive MS are sometimes treated with immunosuppressants, intended to arrest progression by inducing a plateau in deterioration. But these agents, including cyclophosphamide, azathioprine, and cyclosporine, have been used with only modest benefits or conflicting outcomes in prospective, double-blind, controlled clinical trials. What's more, the hazards of immunosuppressants include infection, bone marrow suppression, sterility, and carcinogenesis. Total lymphoid irradiation is another form of immunosuppression that has been shown to slow chronic progressive MS; however, its benefits are related to the level of immune system destruction. Since radiation has no dose-threshold for neoplasia, the long-term effects of total lymphoid irradiation are unknown.

Systemic Oral Enzymes Offer Real Hope for MS Patients
Over 20 years ago Dr. Max Wolf, the originator of systemic oral enzyme therapy, reported of his frequent success in achieving remissions in intermittent MS by administering Wobenzym® N.

These initial results were confirmed by Dr. Neuhofer who repeatedly published her own extensive therapeutic experiences using Wobenzym N. In an early report of results among 150 of her patients, chronic MS was evident in 107 and intermittent progression in 43. A substantial improvement took place in 45 of the patients with chronic progressive MS. Twenty-six remained stabled, twelve suffered further deterioration, and 24 discontinued therapy generally because of the cost of the systemic oral enzymes, or due to difficulties with the family doctor. But for the most part, patients with intermittent progression responded substantially better to enzyme therapy than if they had only been using conventional therapy, according to the doctor's observations. In fact, distinct improvement was evident in 35 of the 43 patients. If prophylactic enzyme therapy began between episodic intervals, the patients either remained free of recurrences or the periods of remission were maintained substantially longer.[124, 125, 126]

We have further clinical validation. In 1992, assistant professor Ulf Baumhackl, chief physician of the neurological department of the hospital in St. Pölten, Austria, reported the results of his investigations at a meeting of the International Neurological Society held in Bad Ischel, Austria.[127] Following a therapeutic and observation period of two years, and taking the symptoms of the illness into consideration, the patients who had received enzymes demonstrated substantially better improvements than those patients who had been treated with cortisone and/or cytostatics.

Professor Kretschowa, a full professor of neurology at the University of Prague, Czechia, also carried out an open clinical

How Enzymes Protect the Myelin Sheath

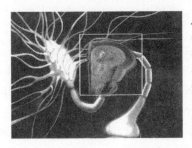

A healthy nerve cell with endings (axons). The coating of the nerve filaments contains periodic constrictions known as the node's of Ranvier which enable a more rapid conduction of the nervous impulse. The enlargement reveals a cross section of the nerve fiber and this coating.

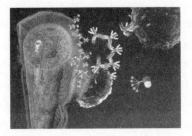

Immune complexes and autoantibodies are bonded to the myelin sheath of the nerve fibers. Complement proteins accumulate (to form complexes) and subsequently activate the complement cascade. With the aid of adhesion molecules, a special, sensitized, cytoclastic T lymphocyte attempts to dock onto the myelin sheath. This myelin sheath is inflamed and larger segments have already been destroyed.

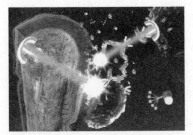

Enzymes break down the immune complexes and autoantibodies. They thereby reduce the complement reaction and prevent consequent destruction of the myelin sheath. The adhesion molecules of the cytoclastic lymphocytes are altered to such an extent that the accumulation of these cells within the myelin sheath does not take place. Enzymes are unable to repair the damage which has already occurred, but the extent of the inflammation can be reduced.

study on the enzyme therapy of MS patients. After two years of therapy, she was able to demonstrate the substantial advantages of enzyme therapy as compared with the combined treatment of cortisone and azathioprine therapy in the treatment of all symptoms of multiple sclerosis.

A large-scale, multi-center study performed at a number of neurological clinics was performed in order to investigate the limits of enzyme therapy in detail. Here, those physicians who have already obtained extensive experience with enzyme therapy are of the opinion that such a treatment with enzymes can help to improve the destiny of MS patients.

Currently a multi-center placebo-controlled clinical trial, which involves 23 neurological treatment centers all over Europe, has been recently completed. Presently the biomedical evaluation is ongoing. The first results will be available soon. What we do know is that enzymes have substantial advantages over the latest medical drug of choice, interferon ß, because they have much less side effects, they are much cheaper and can be used over very long periods. In some MS patients, resistance against interferon ß develops after three to six month of treatment. If the results from the multi-center trial turn out to be as positive as the Neuhofer results, this would be a major improvement in the treatability of MS.

As with juvenile diabetes, funding of such studies should be a public imperative, both in Europe and North America.

Fibrocystic Breast Disease

Diseases of the female breast play a predominant role in women's health care. Although these diseases are often benign, they may nonetheless be uncomfortable. Often, fibrocystic breast disease occurs in relation to menstruation in younger women and is accompanied by varying pain severity.

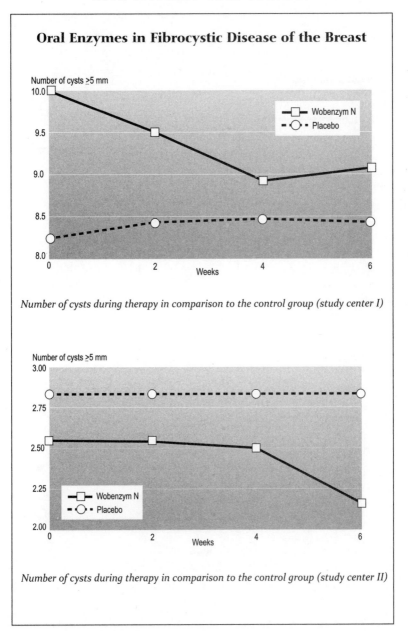

Oral Enzymes in Fibrocystic Disease of the Breast

Number of cysts ≥5 mm

Number of cysts during therapy in comparison to the control group (study center I)

Number of cysts ≥5 mm

Number of cysts during therapy in comparison to the control group (study center II)

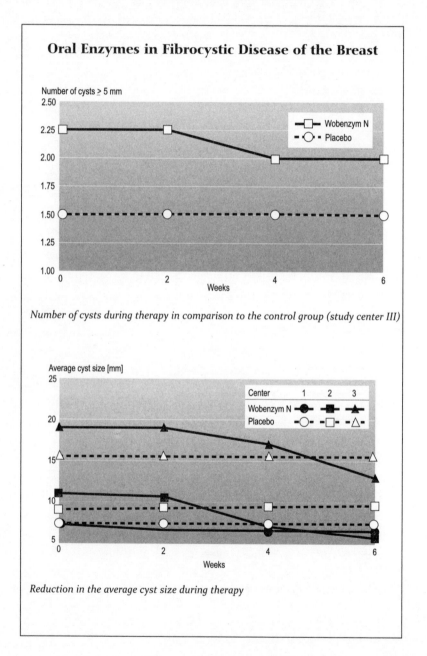

Oral Enzymes in Fibrocystic Disease of the Breast

Number of cysts during therapy in comparison to the control group (study center III)

Reduction in the average cyst size during therapy

In one study, 124 women received ten coated tablets of Wobenzym N twice daily while another 123 women received Wobenzym N together with 1,000 mg of vitamin E. The therapeutic success of the regimen was based on sensation of breast pain and tenderness and via use of advanced non-radiation imaging techniques.[129, 130]

After six weeks of treatment, 80 of the patients in the Wobenzym N group were free of complaints. The proportion of patients free of complaints increased to 85% under the combined regimen of Wobenzym N and vitamin E. Subjective freedom from complaints also was noted significantly earlier.

Although some cases recurred after one to six months, these responded promptly to renewed therapy. Due to the tendency to recurrence, it is recommended that both preparations be used as maintenance therapy.[130]

In another study, the benefits of Wobenzym N were examined in a six-week randomized, placebo-controlled, double-blind multisite study. Ninety-six patients with breast disease including cysts, verified by mammography, took part.[131] Both groups of 48 patients each received ten coated tablets of Wobenzym N or placebo twice daily. Prior to treatment, complaints such as pressure, tension and swelling had persisted for an average of 17.5 days in the Wobenzym N group and an average of 16.2 days in the placebo group.

Following treatment, whereas only insignificant changes were found in the placebo group, a significant reduction in the diameter of cysts took place in the group receiving the Wobenzym N preparation. Intensity of complaints was also reduced substantially.

In the Wobenzym N group, 19 patients complained of unpleasant symptom in the gastrointestinal tract. Only three patients discontinued the therapy for this reason. Nine of the patients in the placebo group complained of adverse effects and two of them discontinued therapy. Three patients of the placebo group discontinued therapy due to its inefficacy.

How to Use Wobenzym N for Fibrocystic Breast Disease

Take ten Wobenzym N tablets twice daily 35 to 45 minutes before meals and 1,000 mg of vitamin E with meals. Continue with a maintenance dose of three to five tablets three times daily with 400 to 600 mg of vitamin E.

13
How to Use
Systemic Oral Enzymes

Why do so many tablets have to be taken? Sensibly, many of us share an aversion against taking tablets. This is especially pronounced in cases where "exorbitant quantities" have to be swallowed, for example, when using systemic oral enzymes in the treatment of injuries and other acute or stubborn chronic conditions. Why are such quantities mandatory in systemic oral enzyme therapy?

It is very difficult to pack a sufficient amount of enzyme molecules into a tablet. In order to maintain their activity, the manufacture of tablets with enzymes requires special care; similar to the packaging of porcelain vases, each molecule must, more or less, be packaged individually. This "packaging material," as well as the acid-resistant covering of the enteric-coated tablets, requires space.

Furthermore, as can be seen in the example which follows, the enzyme molecules themselves are also very large. The enzyme trypsin has a molecular weight of approximately 24,000, Daltons whereas that of acetylsalicylic acid (aspirin) is only about 200 Daltons. Both molecules are composed primarily of the elements carbon, hydrogen and oxygen and therefore have a comparable mass density. If the acetylsalicylic acid molecule were 200 times larger, that is if it were as large as trypsin enzyme, it would be necessary to take approximately 200 tablets.

Individual Dosing

Enzyme molecules are resorbed by the intestines through the use of special transport mechanisms. This active performance by the intestinal cells is highly dependent on individual factors and on the actual conditions in the intestines of the individual. Suggested dosages can therefore represent only rough guidelines. Initially, the enzyme dosage should be relatively high and subsequently reduced step by step until the individual maintenance dose has been reached.

In order to obtain the best level of enzyme concentration balanced over the day, it is recommended that the dosage be given in three or more divided individual doses. Thus, it is better to take five tablets three times a day in three or more divided doses than a single dose of 15 tablets. The exception to this would be highly painful acute conditions such as following sports injuries, in which case a massive–dose therapy protocol of 15 to 20 tablets several times daily is indicated.

Administration should be carried out 30 minutes to one hour before or at least one to two hours after a meal. It is important that the enzyme preparation always be taken with a sufficient amount of water (at least one eight–ounce glass).

The usual maintenance dose is three to five tablets two to three times daily. However, many doctors experienced with enzymes find that their patients receive even better results with dosages of five to ten tablets three times daily.

Side Effects

Enzyme combination preparations have undergone extensive toxicological investigations. Neither toxic effects to users or the fetus have been seen. Although the German Health Service Authorities recorded the prescription of 1.4 million of these enzyme combination preparations in 1992, there were no reports of any grave adverse effects.

Even when given at high doses and for longer periods of time, proteolytic enzymes are seen to be nearly free of side effects. Minor allergic reactions (reddening of the skin) were rarely observed, although these symptoms disappeared completely after discontinuing the enzyme therapy.

A harmless alteration in the consistency, color and odor of the stool may occur, but this is of little consequence. Gastrointestinal disturbances like a feeling of fullness, flatulence or nausea, as well as diarrhea may also be seen in individual cases. Relief from these symptoms can be attained by distributing the daily dosage in the form of numerous individual dosages throughout the day. Discontinuing therapy is only necessary on very rare occasions.

Who Should Not Take Advantage of Systemic Oral Enzyme Therapy?

❖ Individuals who tend to suffer from allergies, especially allergies to proteins, should generally avoid the administration of enzyme preparations.

❖ Enzyme preparations should be discontinued approximately 24 hours before undergoing operative surgery which might involve a great loss of blood.

❖ The use of these products should also be avoided by Individuals with congenital disturbances in coagulation or with coagulatory disturbances which have developed in the course of advanced liver or kidney disease.

❖ The concomitant use of anticoagulants (e.g., dicumarol) may make an alteration in their dosage mandatory.

❖ Pharmaceuticals which inhibit platelet aggregation (e.g., aspirin) may demonstrate a stronger effect, thereby requiring enzyme users to work with their doctor to lower the dosage of their medication.

❖ Every pharmaceutical therapy must be evaluated critically during pregnancy. This is especially true during the first and last third of the pregnancy. Use enzymes only under the guidance of a qualified health professional.

Why Wobenzym° N

In this detailed report, I have told you about one of the most powerful drug-free healing systems now available to health-conscious consumers who are seeking alternatives to potentially toxic prescription and over-the-counter painkillers.

Furthermore, enzymes have many other important health benefits, including maintaining circulatory health and in many other diverse inflammatory conditions, as well as synergizing effects of medically necessary drugs.

However, I have to stress that virtually all of the studies performed on systemic oral enzymes were done with the Wobenzym N or other Mucos Pharma systemic oral enzyme formulas. Other companies have used these studies to support their formulas, but their formulas cannot produce the same results as Wobenzym N. There are key manufacturing practices utilized by Mucos Pharma GmbH of Germany to produce Wobenzym N, including stability and activity of the actual enzymes. Wobenzym N is the only enzyme product in America measured in F.I.P. units, the international standard of measurement for actual enzyme activity. Most other enzyme products are measured only by their weight and cannot guarantee the actual activity of the enzymes.

Wobenzym N is the most thoroughly researched enzyme mixture available worldwide. Wobenzym N contains five potent enzymes including pancreatin, trypsin, chymotrypsin, brome-lain, and papain, as well as the bioflavonoid rutin.

Wobenzym N is clearly the most scientifically and clinically validated enzyme formula in the world. This is simply a fact. Also, the research into Wobenzym N continues to mount and be updated, confirmed, revalidated, explored.

Enzymes are not as fast acting as typical NSAIDs such as ibuprofen, but over the long run, they are much safer and more effective.

14
Seeking Salubrity—
A State of Enviable Health

M y hope is that you seek salubrity—an ancient Greek word that means a state of enviable health. The information contained here should give you a basis for doing so without the drawbacks of side effects and toxicities so often seen with aggressive polypharmacy.

Modern medicine, with all its advances, has not found the perfect procedure or the safe pill. Our bodies seek health. We don't usually crave poisons. Through nutrition, sensible exercise, and a healthy positive attitude, we can make changes that will improve our health. The result will be a fuller and more productive life.

Are you up to the challenge? Do you want to do more? Learn how to get better? Become who you were always meant to be?

You chose to come through the door with us by reading this book. Now get healthy. Find salubrity!

15

Resources

Wobenzym N® is distributed in the United States by the premiere whole foods nutrition company Garden of Life.
• www.gardenoflife.com
   Find more enzyme–related articles at www.healthylivingmag.com and www.systemicenzymesupport.org

Social Media
• www.twitter.com/whywobenzym **twitter**

How to Find a Physician Who Practices Complementary Medicine
To find a physician visit either www.freedompressonline.com or contact the American College for Advancement in Medicine, 8001 Irvine Center Drive, Suite 825, Irvine, California 92618, website: www.acam.org or call (800) 532-3688.

Appendix 1

A Balanced View of Aspirin

In the late 1940s, Glendale physician Lawrence Craven started advising his male patients to take aspirin. It was a complete break from medical tradition. The doctor's patients were not using aspirin to relieve mild pain, reduce fever, or curb inflammation associated with conditions like rheumatoid arthritis. Rather, they were taking one of the little white pills everyday to prevent heart attacks.

Dr. Craven's advice was based on a prior observation: if tonsillectomy patients were given aspirin they continued to bleed, leading him to speculate aspirin had an anti-clotting effect on blood. Since heart attacks are caused by clotting, Craven reasoned, a substance that prevented this phenomenon could possibly prevent heart attacks.

By 1950, some 400 men were using aspirin on the doctor's advice. None had suffered heart attacks. By 1956, no heart attacks had occurred among 8,000 men now using aspirin.

Yet, as so often happens, these findings were greeted with little note and even hostility by the medical community, notes Joe Graedon, author of *The Aspirin Handbook*.

"The medical community, for the most part, seemed oblivious, if not antagonistic," Graedon told *The Los Angeles Times* in a September 29, 1994 report. "If only we would have paid attention to Dr. Craven. . . . Tens of thousands, perhaps hundreds of thousands, of lives were lost while we sat on our hands."

Yet, in a sense, medical science has moved extraordinarily quickly to embrace aspirin since Dr. Craven's first reports in the late 1940s and 1950s, and the little white pill that costs at most only pennies a day to take continues to make news. In March 1995, the *Harvard Health Letter* ranked aspirin among the top ten medical advances of 1994 for its ability to decrease blood clots and, therefore, heart attacks, noting nearly everyone who has ever had a heart attack or stroke, suffers from angina, or has undergone coronary artery bypass surgery should take one-half to one aspirin tablet daily unless they are allergic to the drug. "Worldwide adoption of this advice by these and other high-risk patients would prevent about 100,000 deaths and twice as many nonfatal strokes and heart attacks each year," reports the *Harvard Health Letter*. Moreover, aspirin can reduce the risk of a first heart attack, in both men and women. In the August 1991 *Circulation*, P.M. Ridker and co-investigators reported results from a randomized, double-blind placebo-controlled trial of alternate-day aspirin use among 22,071 U.S. male physicians who were followed for 60.2 months, reporting alternate-day aspirin therapy significantly reduced the risk of a first myocardial infarction. In the July 24–31, 1991 *Journal of the American Medical Association* (JAMA), J.E. Manson and co-investigators reported results, from a study of 87,678 registered nurses in 11 U.S. states, in which it was found that the use of one through six aspirin per week appeared to be associated with a reduced risk of a first heart attack among women.

To reach even this medically historic point, however, required literally thousands of years. "About 3500 years ago the Ebers papyrus recommended the application of a decoction of the dried leaves of Myrtle to the abdomen and back to expel rheumatic pains from the womb. A thousand years later Hippocrates championed the juices of the Poplar tree for treating eye diseases and those of Willow bark for pain in childbirth and for fever. All contain salicylates," note J.R. Vane and R.M. Botting in *Aspirin and Other Salicylates.*

The history of modern aspirin dates back about a century. In 1899, a product containing a synthetic version of salicylic acid, acetylsalicylic acid, began to be marketed as an "over-the-counter" pain killer by the Bayer Company of Germany. The name aspirin was based on the fact that it contained the root of *Spiraea ulmeria* (queen of the meadow plant, a natural source of salicylic acid), together with an "A" as an abbreviation for "acetyl," note Vane and Botting. Aspirin was accepted into the German Pharmacopoeia that year. Bayer soon began marketing its product in the United States.

Yet for all of its popularity, the medical community did not begin to understand how aspirin exerts its powerful effects on human health until the 1960s and 1970s. In essence, aspirin is a broad-spectrum inhibitor of prostaglandins, a family of fatty acids so ubiquitous in the human body they are detected in almost every tissue and body fluid. First discovered in the 1930s, prostaglandins produce a wide range of effects embracing practically every biological function, note Vane and Botting. However, as the *Los Angeles Times* report notes, "excess prostaglandin can cause headaches, fever and arthritis inflammation, as well as production of blood clots that lead to cardiovascular disease. Tumor cells, particularly in colon cancer, have high levels of prostaglandins." Prostaglandins also are potent inducers of fever and inflammation. Not surprisingly, pain can be lessened by suppressing the formation of certain prostaglandins. In 1971, according to *Aspirin and Other Salicylates*, Vane and his colleagues at the

Royal College of Surgeons of England discovered aspirin inhibits the formation of prostaglandins.

Beyond studies exploring aspirin's role in reducing cardiovascular disease, research has spilled over into other areas of human health. The studies on aspirin's additional alleged health benefits, however, have not always shown ironclad proof of health benefits. Among additional areas of research:

Cataract prevention. Some researchers' studies have raised the question of a possible benefit of aspirin on the prevention of cataract, a potentially blinding opacity of the eye's lens, note J.M. Seddon and co-investigators in the February 1991 *Archives of Ophthalmology.* In their own analysis of data collected from the Physicians' Health Study involving 22,071 male physicians, aged 40 to 84 years, who were taking 325 milligrams (mg) of aspirin on alternate days, the researchers found a small, nonsignificant reduction of cataracts in those physicians using aspirin compared to those who were not. Overall, Seddon and co-investigators note alternate-day aspirin therapy may have a possible but small benefit.

Colorectal cancer prevention. A Harvard University study of some 47,900 male health professionals found a 32 percent risk reduction among those taking aspirin at least twice a week, reports *The Los Angeles Times.* However, in the August 4, 1993 *Journal of the National Cancer Institute,* P.H. Gann and co-investigators noted their analysis of data, derived from the Physicians' Health Study, demonstrated that taking aspirin, at a dose adequate for preventing heart attacks, was not associated with a significant reduction in the incidence of colo-rectal cancer.

Reducing severity of Alzheimer's disease. Noting that evidence of inflammation has been found in the brain tissue of patients with Alzheimer's disease, researchers have speculated whether aspirin or other stronger versions of aspirin known as nons-

teroidal anti–inflammatory drugs (NSAIDs) could slow its progression. In a study published in the January 1995 Neurology,
J.B. Rich and co–investigators at Johns Hopkins University
reviewed the records of 209 patients with Alzheimer's disease.
Some 32 of them had taken either aspirin or other NSAIDs
during the last year. The patients underwent extensive neu-
ropsychologic testing initially and one year later. After adjust-
ing for duration of Alzheimer's disease, the aspirin–NSAID
users had significantly better scores than other patients on a
variety of mental acuity tests. During a year of follow–up, the
NSAID–aspirin group also had smaller declines on several test
scores compared with controls. In a related finding, Dr. Patrick
McGeer, of the University of British Columbia, observed that
people with rheumatoid arthritis, who use aspirin against
joint inflammation, appear to suffer much less frequently from
Alzheimer's disease. "It was my hope that you might be able
to treat Alzheimer's disease just by going into your local
supermarket and buying bottles of aspirin," McGeer told *The
Los Angeles Times*. "But then we realized we were going to have
to give doses that would be beyond what could safely be
taken on a casual basis." However, McGeer subsequently discovered a stronger NSAID, indomethacin, has shown evidence
of completely halting progression of the disease, notes the *Los
Angeles Times*.

Migraine prevention. Aspirin's use for the prevention of recur-
ring migraine headaches appears promising. In the October 3,
1990 JAMA, J.E. Buring and co–investigators reported a significant 20 percent reduction in migraine recurrence rate among
men using aspirin compared to those who did not, based on
results from the Physicians' Health Study. In the January 30, 1988
British Medical Journal Clinical Research Edition, R. Peto and co-

investigators reported, in a six-year randomized trial conducted among 5,139 apparently healthy male doctors, men taking 500 mg aspirin daily had significantly less migraines than in the control group.

As for its traditional usage in relieving mild to moderate pain and reducing fever and inflammation, aspirin continues to impress the medical community, notes Sidney M. Wolfe, M.D. of the Public Citizen Health Research Group, in Washington, D.C., and co-author of *Worst Pills Best Pills*. "All prescription drugs for rheumatoid arthritis are much more expensive than aspirin, have significant side effects, and are no more than effective than aspirin," says Wolfe. Moreover, although all NSAIDs as well as acetaminophen-containing products (e.g., Tylenol) pose the risk of kidney failure when used excessively and chronically, aspirin is least likely to pose these risks, note T.V. Perneger and co-investigators in the December 22, 1994 *New England Journal of Medicine*.

However, for those men and women over age 70 considering use of aspirin as prophylactic therapy against heart disease, they should think twice about its regular use if they are otherwise at low risk for heart disease or stroke. The danger of bleeding complications may outweigh the benefits. In the July 1993 *Clinical Pharmacology Therapy*, C.A. Silagy and co-investigators observed that in a double-blind, randomized placebo-controlled trial of 400 subjects who were 70 years of age or older, who received either 100 mg of enteric-coated aspirin daily or placebo (and who had no pre-existing major vascular diseases at the time of entry), that there were more gastrointestinal symptoms among those using aspirin and that clinically evident gastrointestinal bleeding occurred in three percent of the subjects receiving aspirin and none receiving placebo. The researchers concluded until the risk-benefit trade-off from the use of low-dose aspirin in the elderly is established with an appropriate clinical trial, caution should be exercised when this compound is used for primary prevention of cardiovascular disease in this age group.

This study points up the recommendation that people should not take aspirin if they have ulcers, a severely irritated stomach, gout, severe anemia, hemophilia or other bleeding problems. "If you take aspirin only occasionally, plain, generic aspirin is best," says Wolfe. For long-term use, Wolfe asserts enterically coated aspirin will help prevent stomach bleeding–(although the July 1993 *Clinical Pharmacology Therapy* report demonstrates even low–dose enterically coated aspirin can cause such bleeding in the elderly). Wolfe recommends against buffered aspirin "since it is no better than plain aspirin and is more costly." Indeed, the July 8, 1977 *Federal Register* notes the findings of a Food and Drug Administration advisory committee that found no credible evidence buffered aspirin is gentler to the stomach than regular aspirin.

There is also a small increased risk when taking aspirin for the most serious kinds of disabling strokes that occur, not from blood clots, but from hemorrhage. In a May 15, 1991, report in the *Annals of Internal Medicine*, P.M. Ridker and co–investigators noted their results, although based on small numbers, suggested an apparent increase in frequency of stroke with aspirin therapy. These results confirmed the 1988 report in the *British Medical Journal Clinical Research Edition*. In this case, the reduction in non-fatal strokes was a substantial 25 percent, but disabling strokes were somewhat commoner among those given aspirin. Thus, the bottom line appears to be aspirin can prevent less serious types of stroke but may increase the risk of those potentially most disabling. (It is especially important that people not use aspirin if they are taking anticoagulant drugs such as heparin or warfarin, notes Wolfe.)

Finally, aspirin should never be given to children under the age of two or under age 16 who are suffering from a cold, flu, or chicken pox because of the risk of Reye's Syndrome, a potentially fatal illness.

The amount to take is also important. One of the nation's leading aspirin researchers, Dr. Charles Hennekens, of Brigham and Women's Hospital in Boston, advises the use of about 80 mg.

Don't take this little white pill without supervision, advises Graedon. "Anyone who is contemplating a lifelong regimen of aspirin needs to be under medical supervision. This is not a do-it-yourself project."

Glossary

Active movements: Movements specifically initiated by the patient.

Amino acids: Any of a class of organic compounds containing at least amino group (derived from ammonia) and used as a building block for protein in the human body.

Analgesic: Pain relief medication, usually without cartilage regenerating properties.

Antibody: Protein molecule produced by the immune system's B cells as a primary immune defense. These combine with antigens to firm circulating immune complexes which can cause inflammation and impair immunity.

Antigen: Substances that stimulates the body's production of antibodies.

Antioxidant: Substance that scavenges free radicals and prevents oxidation of bodily tissues and cells.

Arachidonic acid: A type of prostaglandin found almost entirely in animal foods (along with saturated fat) which can increase the body's inflammation levels.

Arthralgia: Pain in joints.

Arthritis: Inflammation of joints. There are more than 100 types of arthritis.

Articular cartilage: Cushioned, watery, highly slick cartilage in the area of the joints at ends of bones.

Auto–immune: A process by which the body's immune system turns on or attacks the body's own tissues. Rheumatoid arthritis is considered an auto–immune disease.

Bacteria: Microscopic one–celled organisms.

Bioflavonoid: Substances once known as Vitamin P and close-ly related in nature to ascorbic acid. These water–soluble compounds are generally yellow in coloration and found in citrus, rose hips and other plants. Plants richest in bioflavonoids are often most colorful. They are powerful antioxidants and also help to maintain the structure and integrity of the body's collagen.

Bone marrow: Soft, vascular tissue in the cavities of bones where blood cells are formed.

Cartilage: Firm, white–blue substance at ends of bones. Highly water–dependent. Has no blood vessels. Acts as body's shock absorber.

Chondrocytes: The cells in joints that produce the substances that make–up cartilage.

Circulating Immune Complex: A globulin of antibodies and antigens with other tissue matter that is formed during some inflammatory and auto–immune diseases such as rheuma-toid arthritis and may be deposited in the body's tissues, causing intense inflammation.

Collagen: Substance making up body's connective tissues. Collagen gives cartilage its "spring." The collagen found in joints is called Collagen Type II.

Corticosteroid: Powerful steroid medication that reduces inflammation. Complications include damage to heart, bone, immune systems. Inhibits the production of prostaglandins but also white blood cells.

Crepitus: The crackling sound joints make.

Cyst: Sac of fluid that forms in bone as cartilage is worn away.

Duodenal ulcer: A store in the mucous membranes, located in the first portion of the small intestine.

Fascia: A band or sheath of connective tissue covering, supporting, or connecting the muscles or internal organs of the body.

Free Radical: Substance or molecular fragment with one or more unpaired electrons. It is highly reactive, stripping and damaging other cells in a process called oxidation as it searches for an electron match.

Glucosamine: An amino sugar occurring in vertebrate tissues including that of marine shells and other small marine creatures from where it is usually harvested.

Glucosamine sulfate (also spelled sulphate): A specific form of glucosamine used as an osteoarthritis healing agent.

Glycosaminoglycans: A group of polysaccharides that are responsible for water retention in cartilage and are the building blocks of proteoglycans.

Gout: Painful inflammation usually of the big toes, characterized by an excess of uric acid in the blood that leads to crystalline deposits in the small joints.

Health Maintenance Organization (HMO): Organization that delivers medical services to pre-selected care givers at a fixed price on a pre-paid basis.

Herb: A plant valued for its medicinal properties.

Histamine: Derived from the amino acid histidine, histamines are released particularly by damaged mast cells during allergic reactions. They cause dilation and blood vessel permeability and may cause inflammation.

Isometrics: A form of exercise in which immovable pressure is applied, such as pressing hands against each other or neck against hand, or pushing into a wall.

Leukotrienes: Lipid produced by white blood cells in an immune response to antigens that contributes to allergic asthma and inflammatory reactions.

Ligament: Band of strong connective tissue that connects bones and holds organs in place.

NSAIDs: Non Steroidal Anti-inflammatory Agents. Included in this class of agents are aspirin and the many other agents that are inhibitors of the enzyme system(s) called cyclo-oxygenase.

Opioid: Semi-synthetic or synthetic opiumlike substance.

Osteoarthritis: The "wear and tear" or bio-mechanical form of arthritis, as opposed to rheumatoid arthritis, which is an auto-immune disease.

Osteophytes: Mineralized outgrowths of bone in damaged cartilage areas.

Passive movement: Movement initiated or aided by another person.

Prostaglandins: Hormone-like fatty acid substances that influence body's inflammation levels, temperature, muscular contractions and many other functions. As with cholesterol, there are thought to be "good" prostaglandins and "bad" prostaglandins.

Protein: Composed of long chains of amino acids and constituting much of the mass of living organisms.

Proteoglycans: Mortar-like substance made from protein and sugar that are the building blocks of cartilage.

Rheumatoid arthritis: Auto-immune form of arthritis.

Slow Acting Drug in Osteoarthritis: Specific term applied to glucosamine sulfate by the International League Against Rheumatism.

Sulfate: Derived from sulfuric acid and a nutrient for the body's joint matrix and other tissues.

Synovial fluid: A clear, viscous, lubricating main fluid found in joints.

Synovial membrane (also known as synovium): The soft encapsulating material surrounding the joint that allows nutrients and toxins and other liquids to pass in and out.

Tendons: White, fibrous cord or band that connects muscles to bones.

Thromboxane: Substance formed in blood platelets that causes clotting.

Bibliography of Articles on Wobenzym N Available through Medline

PubMed, a free resource developed and maintained by the National Center for Biotechnology Information (NCBI), at the U.S. National Library of Medicine (NLM), located at the National Institutes of Health (NIH), lets you search millions of journal citations and abstracts in the fields of medicine, nursing, dentistry, veterinary medicine, the health care system, and preclinical sciences. It includes access to MEDLINE® and to citations for selected articles in life science journals not included in MEDLINE. References for Wobenzym N are listed in chronological order, starting with the most recent.

1. The influence of enzymes on adhesive processes in the abdominal cavity. Minaev SV, Obozin VS, Barnash GM, Obedin AN. *Eur J Pediatr Surg.* 2009 Dec;19(6):380–3.
2. [Modern approach to the rehabilitation of children with fractured long tubular bones] Isaeva AV, Minaev SV, Sternin IuI, Minaeva NV. *Vopr Kurortol Fizioter Lech Fiz Kult.* 2009 May–Jun;(3):29–31. Russian.
3. [New aspects of pathogenesis of adhesive process in the abdominal cavity] Minaev SV, Obozin VS, Pustoshkina LT, Barnash GM, Tuliubaev IN. *Vestn Khir Im I I Grek.* 2009;168(1):45–9. Russian.
4. Enzymes, trophoblasts, and cancer: the afterlife of an idea (1924–2008). Moss RW. *Integr Cancer Ther.* 2008 Dec;7(4):262–75.

5. [Systemic poly-enzyme therapy in prophylaxis of venous
    blood circulation disorder in the lower limbs in modern
    sport] Sternin IuI, Safonov LV, Levando VA. *Voen Med Zh.*
    2008 May;329(5):42-5. Russian. No abstract available.
6. [Enzyme therapy of patients with pyo-inflammatory disease
    of maxillofacial area] Minaev SV, Ibragimov OR, Zelenskiĭ VA,
    Minaeva NV. *Voen Med Zh.* 2007 Nov;328(11):25-7, 96. Russian.
7. [Antioxidant effect of wobenzym applied for patients with
    chronic glomerulonephritis] Mukhin IV. Lik Sprava. 2007
    Jan-Mar;(1-2):58-61. Ukrainian.
8. [Systemic enzyme therapy in the treatment of children with
    lower orbital wall fractures] Dubovskaia LA, Guseva MR,
    Gorbunova ED, Gorbunov AV, Kazinskaia NV. *Vestn
    Oftalmol.* 2006 Nov-Dec;122(6):20-3. Russian.
9. [Impaired immunological status due to the urogenital chlamydio-
    sis in women of reproductive age and its correction] Tabukashvili
    NG. *Georgian Med News.* 2006 Oct;(139):57-60. Russian.
10. Where do the immunostimulatory effects of oral proteolytic
    enzymes ('systemic enzyme therapy') come from? Microbial
    proteolysis as a possible starting point. Biziulevicius GA.
    Med Hypotheses. 2006;67(6):1386-8. Epub 2006 Jul 25.
11. [Systemic enzymotherapy as a method of prophylaxis of
    postradiation complications in oncological patients]
    Hubarieva HO, Kindzel's'kyĭ LP, Ponomar'ova OV, Udatova
    TV, Shpil'ova SI, Smolanka II, Korovin SI, Ivankin VS.
    Lik Sprava. 2000 Oct-Dec;(7-8):94-100. Ukrainian.
12. [Effects of wobenzyme on certain indices for the oxidation-
    antioxidation homeostasis and erythrocyte morphofunc-
    tional status in elderly and senile patients with peptic ulcer]
    Fediv OI. *Lik Sprava.* 2000 Oct-Dec;(7-8):80-4. Ukrainian.
13. [Polyenzymatic therapy in prevention of adhesive processes
    in the abdominal cavity in children] Minaev SV, Nemilova
    TK, Knorring GIu. *Vestn Khir Im I I Grek.* 2006;165(1):49-54.
    Russian.

14. Wobenzym in treatment of recurrent obstructive bronchitis in children. Lanchava N, Nemsadze K, Chkhaidze I, Kandelaki E, Nareklishvili N. *Georgian Med News*. 2005 Oct;(127):50–3.

15. [A case of an asynchronic triple tumorous disorder: a rectal adenocarcinoma, a carcinoma of the kidney and a prostatic adenocarcinoma—case report] Prosvic P, Brod'ák M, Odrázka K, Morávek P. *Rozhl Chir*. 2005 Jan;84(1):41–5. Czech.

16. [Systemic enzyme therapy of experimental gout glomerulonephritis] Ignatenko GA, Mukhin IV. *Patol Fiziol Eksp Ter*. 2004 Oct–Dec;(4):26–8. Russian.

17. [Proteolytic enzymes as an alternative in comparison with nonsteroidal anti–inflammatory drugs (NSAID) in the treatment of degenerative and inflammatory rheumatic disease: systematic review] Heyll U, Münnich U, Senger V. *Med Klin* (Munich). 2003 Nov 15;98(11):609–15. Review. German.

18. [Experimental evaluation of the wound healing dynamics] Minaev SV. *Vestn Khir Im I I Grek*. 2003;162(4):57–62. Russian.

19. [Experimental systemic enzyme therapy of gouty and primary glomerulonephritis] Mukhin IV, Nikolenko VIu. *Eksp Klin Farmakol*. 2003 Jul–Aug;66(4):32–5. Russian.

20. [Systemic enzyme therapy as a method for potentiation of the effect of antibacterial agents] Remezov AP, Knorring GIu. *Antibiot Khimioter*. 2003;48(3):30–3. Review. Russian. No abstract available.

21. [Treatment of dyslipoproteinemia by systemic enzyme therapy in experimental glomerulonephritis] Mukhin IV. *Patol Fiziol Eksp Ter*. 2002 Oct–Dec;(4):27–8. Russian.

22. [Effects of wobenzyme on the blood proteinase–inhibitory system in elderly and senile patients with gastric and duodenal peptic ulcers] Fediv OI. *Lik Sprava*. 2001 May Jun;(3):130–5. Ukrainian.

23. Bromelain is an accelerator of phagocytosis, respiratory burst and Killing of Candida albicans by human granulocytes and monocytes. Brakebusch M, Wintergerst U, Petropoulou T, Notheis G, Husfeld L, Belohradsky BH, Adam D. *Eur J Med Res.* 2001 May 29;6(5):193–200

24. [Fibronectin content in the urine of patients with chronic glomerulonephritis as a test for the efficiency of treatment] Mukhin IV. *Klin Lab Diagn.* 2001 Apr;(4):53–5. Russian.

25. [The effect of Wobenzym on the atherogenic potential and inflammatory factors at the rehabilitation stage for patients who have had a myocardial infarct] Riabokon' EN, Gavrilenko TI, Kornilina EM, Iakushko LV. *Lik Sprava.* 2000 Jul–Aug;(5):111–4. Russian.

26. [The procedure for treating patients with genital endometriosis] Ventskivs'ka IB. Lik *Sprava.* 2000 Jan–Feb;(1):85–6. Ukrainian.

27. [The dynamics of the humoral immunity indices and of the beta 2-microglobulin level in children with chronic hepatitis] Volosianko AB. *Lik Sprava.* 2000 Mar;(2):67–9.

28. [The use of Wobenzym in the comprehensive treatment of patients with digital flexor tendon injury] Strafun SS, Tovmasian VV. *Klin Khir.* 2000;(4):39–40. Russian.

29. [The adaptational properties and immunoregulatory action of a preparation of proteolytic enzymes in experimental stress] Suzdal'nitskiĭ RS, Levando VA, Emel'ianov BA, Sokolov IaA. *Zh Mikrobiol Epidemiol Immunobiol.* 1999 Sep–Oct;(5):103–6. Russian.

30. [The effect of the preparation Wobenzym on the antioxidant protection indices and on the functional–morphological properties of the erythrocytes in a toxic lesion of the liver] Kolomoiets MIu, Shorikov IeI. *Lik Sprava.* 1999 Jul;(5):124–8. Ukrainian.

31. [The pathogenetic basis for and clinical use of systemic enzyme therapy in traumatology and orthopedics] Neverov VA, Klimov AV. *Vestn Khir Im I I Grek.* 1999;158(1):41–4. Russian.

32. [Systemic enzyme therapy in the treatment of supracondylar fractures of the humerus in children] Gál P, Tecl F, Skotáková J, Mach V. *Rozhl Chir.* 1998 Dec;77(12):574–6. Czech.

33. Orally administered proteases in aesthetic surgery. Dusková M, Wald M. *Aesthetic Plast Surg.* 1999 Jan–Feb;23(1):41–4.

34. [The use of enzymes in treating patients with malignant lymphoma with a large tumor mass] Gubareva AA. *Lik Sprava.* 1998 Aug;(6):141–3. Russian.

35. [Wobenzym in the combined pathogenetic therapy of chronic urethrogenic prostatitis] Martynenko AV. *Lik Sprava.* 1998 Aug;(6):118–20. Russian.

36. [The pharmacological action of wobenzym on blood coagulability] Korpan MI, Korpan NN, Chekman IS, Fialka V. *Lik Sprava.* 1997 Jul–Aug;(4):70–2. Russian. No abstract available

37. [Enzyme therapy in the treatment of lymphedema in the arm after breast carcinoma surgery] Adámek J, Prausová J, Wald M. *Rozhl Chir.* 1997 Apr;76(4):203–4. Czech.

38. Adjuvant therapy with hydrolytic enzymes in recurrent laryngeal papillomatosis. Mudrák J, Bobák L, Sebová I. *Acta Otolaryngol Suppl.* 1997;527:128–30.

39. [Concerning a contaminated drug] Franco Patiño R. *Rev Invest Clin.* 1996 May–Jun;48(3):247. Spanish. No abstract available.

40. [Drug therapy of activated arthrosis. On the effectiveness of an enzyme mixture versus diclofenac] Singer F, Oberleitner H. *Wien Med Wochenschr.* 1996;146(3):55–8. German.

41. [Results of a double–blind, randomized comparative study of Wobenzym–placebo in patients with cervical syndrome] Tilscher H, Keusch R, Neumann K. *Wien Med Wochenschr.* 1996;146(5):91–5. German.

42. [Wobenzyme and diuretic therapy in lymphedema after breast operation] Korpan MI, Fialka V. *Wien Med Wochenschr.* 1996;146(4):67–72; discussion 74. German.

43. [Enzyme therapy in treatment of mastopathy. A randomized double-blind clinical study] Rammer E, Friedrich F. *Wien Klin Wochenschr.* 1996;108(6):180–3. German.

44. [Density of adhesive proteins after oral administration of proteolytic enzymes in multiple myeloma] Sakalová A, Kunze R, Holománová D, Hapalová J, Chorváth B, Mistrík M, Sedlák J. *Vnitr Lek.* 1995 Dec;41(12):822–6. Slovak.

45. [Probable coumarin poisoning upon ingestion of an anti-inflammatory agent] Pérez-Jáuregui J, Escate-Cavero A, Vega-Galina J, Ruiz-Argüelles GJ, Macip-Nieto G. *Rev Invest Clin.* 1995 Jul-Aug;47(4):311–3. Spanish.

46. Stimulation of reactive oxygen species production and cytotoxicity in human neutrophils in vitro and after oral administration of a polyenzyme preparation. Zavadova E, Desser L, Mohr T. *Cancer Biother.* 1995 Summer;10(2):147–52.

47. Proteolytic enzymes and amylase induce cytokine production in human peripheral blood mononuclear cells in vitro. Desser L, Rehberger A, Paukovits W. *Cancer Biother.* 1994 Fall;9(3):253–63.

48. [Perioperative enzyme therapy. A significant supplement to postoperative pain therapy?] Hoernecke R, Doenicke A. *Anaesthesist.* 1993 Dec;42(12):856–61. German.

49. Cytokine synthesis in human peripheral blood mononuclear cells after oral administration of polyenzyme preparations. Desser L, Rehberger A, Kokron E, Paukovits W. *Oncology.* 1993 Nov-Dec;50(6):403–7

50. [The favorable effect of hydrolytic enzymes in the treatment of immunocytomas and plasmacytomas] Sakalová A, Mikulecký M, Holománová D, Langner D, Ransberger K, Stauder G, Mistrík M, Gazová S, Chabronová I, Benzová M, et al. *Vnitr Lek.* 1992 Sep;38(9):921–9. Slovak.

51. [Circulating immune complexes and complement fragment iC3b in chronic polyarthritis during 12 months therapy with oral enzymes in comparison with oral gold] Kullich W, Schwann H. *Wien Med Wochenschr.* 1992;142(22):493–7. German.

52. [Acute circulatory shock following administration of the non–regular enzyme preparation Wobe–Mugos] de Smet PA, Pegt GW, Meyboom RH. *Ned Tijdschr Geneeskd.* 1991 Dec 7;135(49):2341–4. Dutch.

53. [Mexican medicinal plants and Grüninger's diet Documentation No.25] Deplazes G, Hauser SP. *Schweiz Rundsch Med Prax.* 1990 May 29;79(22):706–8. German.

54. Induction of tumor necrosis factor in human peripheral–blood mononuclear cells by proteolytic enzymes. Desser L, Rehberger A. *Oncology.* 1990;47(6):475–7.

55. [Anaphylactic reaction in enzyme therapy of multiple sclerosis] Kiessling WR. *Fortschr Neurol Psychiatr.* 1987 Dec;55(12):385–6. German.

56. [Basic studies on enzyme therapy of immune complex diseases] Steffen C, Menzel J. *Wien Klin Wochenschr.* 1985 Apr 12;97(8):376–85. German.

57. [Enzyme therapy in comparison with immune complex determinations in chronic polyarthritis] Steffen C, Smolen J, Miehlke K, Hörger I, Menzel J. *Z Rheumatol.* 1985 Mar–Apr;44(2):51–6. German.

58. [Intestinal resorption with 3H labeled enzyme mixture (wobenzyme)] Steffen C, Menzel J, Smolen J. *Acta Med Austriaca.* 1979;6(1):13–8. German.

References

1   Lazarou, P., et al. "Incidence of adverse drug reactions in hospital-
    ized patients; meta-analysis of prospective studies." *Journal of the
    American Medical Association,* 1998; 279: 1200–1204.
2   Fries, J., et al. "Adverse drug reactions, surveillance." *Arthritis,
    Rheumatology,* 1991; 34: 1353–1360.
3   "FDA approves new pain-killer for arthritis." Associated Press,
    December 31, 1998.
4   The Associated Press. "Report: Celebrex linked to 10 deaths." April
    20, 1999.
5   Percival, M. *Healthy Answers,* Fall 1997: 4.
6   Brown, R.L., et al. "Chronic opioid analgesic therapy for chronic
    low back pain." *Journal of the American Board of Family Practice,*
    1996; 9(3): 191–204.
7   Wittenberg, R.H., et al. "Injection treatment of non-radicular lum-
    balgia." *Orthopade,* 1997; 26(6): 544–552.
8   O'Brien, M.E. & Hoel, D. "Overpowering pain. A serious problem
    comes out of the closet." *Postgraduate Medicine,* October 1997: 4–10.
9   Ibid.
10 Ibid.
11 Ibid.
12 Ibid.
13 Ibid.
14 Ibid.
15 Ibid.
16 Ibid.
17 Ibid.
18 Ibid.

19 Allen, J.E. "Focus on chronic pain; many specialists, but little relief for most sufferers." *Los Angeles Times*, Monday, March 22, 1999; S-1.

20 *The PDR Family Guide to Prescription Drugs*. Third Edition. Montvale, NJ: Medical Economics, 1995, p. 12, 135, 337, 731.

21 *Physicians' Desk Reference*. Montvale, NJ: Medical Economics, 1997, pp. 2576-2578.

22 Ibid.

23 *The Use of Opioids for the Treatment of Chronic Pain*. A consensus statement from the American Academy of Pain Medicine and American Pain Society, 1997. Call 1-847-375-4731 to obtain the report.

24 Crolle, G. & D'Este, E. "Glucosamine sulfate for the management of arthrosis: a controlled clinical investigation." *Current Medical Research and Opinion*, 1980; 7(2): 104-109.

25 Pujalte, J.M., et al. "Double-blind clinical evaluation of oral glucosamine sulphate in the basic treatment of osteoarthrosis." *Current Medical Research and Opinion*, 1980; 7(2): 110-114.

26 Newman, N.M. & Ling, R.S.M. "Acetabular bone destruction related to non-steroidal anti-inflammatory drugs." *Lancet*, 1985; ii: 11-13

27 Solomobn, L. "Drug induced arthropathy and necrosis of the femoral head." *Journal of Bone and Joint Surgery*, 1973; 55B: 246-251.

28 Ronningen, H. & Langeland, N. "Indomethacin treatment in osteoarthritis of the hip joint." *Acta Orthop Scand*, 1979; 50: 169-174.

29 Müller-Fabender, H., et al. "Glucosamine sulfate compared to ibuprofen in osteoarthritis of the knee." Osteoarthritis and Cartilage, 1994; 2: 61-69.

30 Spencer-Green, G. "Drug treatment of arthritis. Update on conventional and less conventional methods." *Postgraduate Medicine*, 1993; 93(7): 129-140.

31 Kremer, J.M. "Severe rheumatoid arthritis: current options in drug therapy." *Geriatrics*, 1990; 45(12): 43-48.

32 "Anti-Inflammatory Drug Wins Approval from FDA." *The Wall Street Journal*. July 7, 1997: B7.

33 Clayman, C. [medical editor]. *The American Medical Association Family Medical Guide*. New York, NY: Random House: 1994, p. 589.

34 Clayman, C., op. cit., p. 590.

35 The Burton Goldberg Group. *Alternative Medicine: The Definitive Guide*. Puyallup, WA: Future Medicine Publishing, Inc., p. 531.

36 Clayman, C., op. cit., p. 590.

37 Murray, M.T. & Pizzorno, J.E. *Encyclopedia of Natural Medicine*, Rocklin, CA: Prima Publishing, 1991.

38 Clayman, C., op. cit., p. 588.

39 Clayman, C., op. cit., p. 588.

40 Steffen, C., et al. "Enzymtherapie im vergleich mit immunkomplexbestimmungen bei chronischer polyarthritis." *Zeitschr. f. Rheumatologie*, 1985; 44: 51.

41 Streichhan, P., et al. "Resorption partikulärer und makromolekularer Darminhaltsstoffe." *Nature- und Ganzheitsmedizin*, 1988; 1: 90.

42 Miehlke, K. "Enzymtherapie bei rheumatoider arthritis." *Nature- und Ganzheitsmedizin*, 1988; 1: 108.

43 Singer, F. "Aktivierte arthrosen knorpelschonend behandeln." In': *Medizinische Enzym-Forschungsgesellschaft* e.V. (ed.): Systemische Enzymtherapie, 10th Symposium, Frankfurt, 1990.

44 Mazurov, V.I., et al. "Systemic enzyme therapy in combination therapy for rheumatic disease." *Oral Enzyme Therapy. Compendium of Results from Clinical Studies with Oral Enzyme Therapy.* Second Russian Symposium, St. Petersburg, Russia, 1996, pp. 15–24.

45 Shaikov, A.V., et al. "Wobenzym in combination therapy for juvenile chronic arthritis." *Oral Enzyme Therapy. Compendium of Results from Clinical Studies with Oral Enzyme Therapy.* Second Russian Symposium, St. Petersburg, Russia, 1996, pp. 28–32.

46 Baici, A., et al. "Analysis of glycosaminoglycans in human serum after oral administration of chondroitin sulfate." *Rheumatology International*, 1992; 12: 81–88.

47 Pipitone, V.R. "Chondroprotection with chondroitin sulfate." Drugs in Experimental and Clinical Research, 1991; 17(1): 3–7.

48 Mazières, B., et al. "Le chondroitin sulfate dayns le traitement de la gonarthrose et de la coxarthrose." *Rev. Rheum. Mal Ostéoartic*, 1992; 59(7–8): 466–472.

49 Morreale P., et al. "Comparison of the antiinflammatory efficacy of chondroitin sulfate and diclofenac sodium in patients with knee osteoarthritis." *Journal of Rheumatology*, 1996 Aug, 23(8):1385–1391.

50 Busci, L., et al. "Efficacy and tolerability of 2 x 400 mg oral chondroitin sulfate as a single dose in the treatment of knee osteoarthritis." In: *Osteoarthritis and Cartilage*, vol. 5, Supp. A, Philadelphia, PA: W.B. Saunders, 1997.

51 Bourgeois, P., et al. "Efficacy and tolerability of chondroitin sulfate 12–mg/day vs. chondroitin sulfate 3 x 400 mg /day vs. placebo." In: *Osteoarthritis and Cartilage*, vol. 5, Supp. A, Philadelphia, PA: W.B. Saunders, 1997.

52 Fleisch, A.M., et al. "A one-year randomized, double-blind, place-
    bo-controlled study with oral chondroitin sulfate in patients with
    knee osteoarthritis." In: *Osteoarthritis and Cartilage*, vol. 5, Supp. A,
    Philadelphia, PA: W.B. Saunders, 1997.

53 Uebelhart, D., et al. "Chondroitin 4 & 6 sulfate. A symptomatic
    slow-acting drug for osteoarthritis, does also have structural mod-
    ifying properties." In: *Osteoarthritis and Cartilage*, vol. 5, Supp. A,
    Philadelphia, PA: W.B. Saunders, 1997.

54 DeLuca, H.F. & Zierold, C. "Mechanisms and functions of vitamin
    D." *Nutr Rev*, 56(2 Pt 2):S4–10; discussion S 54–75.

55 Oelzner, P., et al. "Relationship between disease activity and serum
    levels of vitamin D metabolites and PTH in rheumatoid arthritis."
    Calcif Tissue Int, 1998; 62(3): 193–8.

56 Wordsworth, B.P., et al. "Metabolic bone disease among in-patients
    with rheumatoid arthritis." *Br J Rheumatol*, 1984; 23(4): 251–7.

57 Scott, D.L. et al. "Serum calcium levels in rheumatoid arthritis." *Ann
    Rheum Dis*, 1981; 40(6): 580–3.

58 Stone, J., et al. "Inadequate calcium, folic acid, vitamin E, zinc, and
    selenium intake in rheumatoid arthritis patients: results of a
    dietary survey." *Semin Arthritis Rheum*, 1997; 27(3): 180–5.

59 Vainio, H. & Morgan, G. "Aspirin for the second hundred years:
    new uses for an old drug." *Pharmacol Toxicol*, 1997; 81(4): 151–2.

60 Mazurov, V.I., et. al., op. cit.

61 Ibid.

62 Heidland, A., et al. "Renal fibrosis: role of impaired proteolysis and
    potential therapeutic strategies." *Kidney International*, 1997; Suppl
    62: S32–35.

63 Houston, L. "Dietary change in arthritis." *The Practitioner*, June 1994;
    238: 443–448.

64 Goebel, K.M. "Enzymtherapie bei spondylitis ankylosans." In:
    Medizinische Enzym-Forschungsgesellschaft e.V. (ed.): Systemische
    Enzymtherapie, 17th Symposium, Vienna, 1991.

65 Chappa-Alvarez, R. "Pankreatitisbehandlung mit Wobenzym®."
    Publication in preparation, 1992.

66 Guggenbichler, J.P. "Einfluß hydrolytischer Enzyme auf
    Thrombusbildung und Thrombolyse." *Die Medizinische Welt*, 1988;
    39: 277.

67 Kleine, M.-W. & Pabst, H. "Die wirkung einer oralen enzymthera-
    pie aud experimentell erzeugte hämatome." *Forum des Prakt. Und
    Allgemeinarztes*, 1988; 27: 42.

68   MUCOS: MUCOS–Präparate in der Zahnheilkunde. MUCOS Information, 1980.

69   Vinzenz, K. "Ödembehandlung bei zahnchirurgischen eingriffen mit hydrolytischen enzymen." *Die Quintessenz*, 1991; 7: 1053.

70   Werk, W. "Polyenzympräparat zur Beschleunigung der Narbenbildung." *Proktologie*, 1979(3).

71   Rahn, H.–D. "Wobenzym® nach Gefäßbypassoperationen am bein." In: *Medizinische Enzymforschungsgesellschaft e.V.* (ed.): *Systemische Enzymtherapie*, 17th Symposium, Vienna, 1991.

72   Carillo, A.R. "Klinische untersuchung eines enzymatischen entzündungshemmers in der unfallchirurgie." *Ärztl. Praxis*, 1972; 24: 2307.

73   Rahn, H.–D. & Kilic, M. "Die wirksamkeit hydrolytischer enzyme in der traumatologie. Ergebnise nach 2 prospektiven randomisierten doppelblindstudien." *Allgemeinarzt*, 1990; 19: 178.

74   Rahn, H.D. "Efficacy of hydrolytic enzymes in surgery." In: G.P.H. Hermans, W.L. Mosterd (ed.): *Sports, Medicine and Health*. Amsterdam–New York–Oxford: Excerpta Medica, 1990: 1134.

75   Schwinger: "Wobenzym® bei der behandlung von knie– und sprunggelenksoperationen." Publication

76   Rahn, H.–D., Kilic, M. "Die wirksamkeit hydrolytischer enzyme in der traumatologie. Erggbnise nach 2 prospektiven randomisierten doppelblindstudien." *Allgemeinarzt*, 1990; 19: 178.

77   Rahn, H.–D. "Enzyme verkürzen rekonvaleszenz." In: *Medizinische Enzym-Forschungsgesellschaft*. E.V. (eds.): *Systemische Enzymtherapie*, 13th Symposium, Lindau, 1990.

78   Rahn, H.–D. "Wobenzym® begleitend bei arthroskopischer meniskektomie." Publication in preparation.

79   Guggenbichler, J.P. "Einflub hydrolytischer enzyme auf thrombusbildung und thrombolyse." *Die Medizinische Welt*, 1988; 39: 277

80   Klein M.–W., H. Pabst. "Die wirkung einer oralen enzymtherapie auf experimentell erzeugte hämatome." *Forum des Prakt. Und Allgemeinarztes*, 1988; 27: 42.

81   Inderst, R. "Enzymtherapie–grundlagen und anwendungsmöglichkeiten." *Natur und Ganzheitsmedizin*, 1991(3).

82   Baumüller, M. "Der einsatz von hydrolytischen enzymen bei stumpfen weichteilverletzungen und sprunggelenksdistorsionen." *Allgemeinmedizin* 1990; 19: 178.

83   Kleine, M.–W. & Pabst, H., op. cit.

84   Müller-Hepburn, W. "Anwendung von enzymen in der sportmedizin." *Forum d. Prakt. Arztes*, 1970, 18.

85 Ibid.

86 Baumüller, M. "Der einsatz von hydrolytischen enzymen bei stumpfen weichteilverletzungen und sprunggelenksdistorsionen." *Allgemeinmedizin*, 1990; 19: 178.

87 Blonstein, J.L. "Oral enzyme tablets in the treatment of boxing injuries." *The Practitioner*, April 1967, 198: 547.

88 Ibid.

89 Hiss, W.F. "Enzyme in der sport- und unfallmedizin." *Continuing Education Seminars*, 1979.

90 Boyne, P.S. & Medhurt, H. "Oral anti-inflammatory enzyme therapy in injuries in professional footballers." April 1967, 198: 543.

91 Wörschhauser, S. "Konservative therapie der sportverletungen. Enzympräparate für therapie und prophylaxe." *Allgemeinmedizin*, 1990; 19: 173.

92 Baumüller, M. "Enzyme zur wiederherstellung nach sprungge-lenkdistorsionen." *Z. Allg. Med.*, 1992; 68: 61.

93 Ibid.

94 Baumüller, M. "Therapy of ankle joint distortions with hydrolytic enzymes–results from a double blind clinical trial." In: G.P.H. Hermans, W.L. Mosterd (eds.): *Sports, Medicine and Health*. Excerpta Medica. Amsterdam, New York, Oxford, 1990: 1137.

95 Dzhak, F.W. "Use of Wobenzym" in the treatment of muscle dam-age in athletes." Presented at Second Russian Symposium on Oral Enzyme Therapy, St. Petersburg, Russia, 1996, p. 65–67.

96 Bucci, L.R. *Nutrition Applied to Injury Rehabilitation and Sports Medicine*, Boca Raton: CRC Press, 1995. p. 170.

97 Maseri, A. "Inflammation, atherosclerosis, and ischemic events–exploring the hidden side of the moon." *The New England Journal of Medicine*, 1997; 336(14): 1014–1016.

98 Ridker, P.M., et al. "Inflammation, aspirin, and the risk of cardio-vascular disease in apparently healthy men." *The New England Journal of Medicine*, 1997; 336(14): 973–979, 1014–1016.

99 "Inflammation & the heart." *Nutrition Action Health Letter*, June, 1997: 14.

100 Maseri, A., op. cit.

101 Leskovar, P. "AIDS: Neuartige therapiekonzepte." *Dtsch. Zeitschr. Onkol*, 1990; 2.

102 Rosanova, A. "Der gegenwärtige stand der enzymtherapie bei malignen tumoren." *Arzt. Praxis*, 1974; 16: 1442.

103   Wolf, M. & Ransberger, K. *Enzymtherapie.* Vienna: Maudrich Verlag, 1970.

104   "Inflammation & the heart." *Nutrition Action Health Letter,* June, 1997: 14.

105   Kunze, R. Unpublished *in vivo* studies, personal communication, October 14, 1997.

106   Vinzenz, K., op.cit.

107   Sledsewskaja, I.K., et al. "Wobenzym® administration in patients after myocardial infarction." *Oral Enzyme Therapy. Compendium of Results from Clinical Studies with Oral Enzyme Therapy.* Second Russian Symposium, St. Petersburg, Russia, 1996, pp. 90–92.

108   Inderst, R. "Enzymtherapie–grundlagen und anwen- dungsmöglichkeiten." *Naturund Ganzheitsmedizin,* 1991; 3.

109   Grimminger, A. "Enzymtherapie bei thoraxerkrankungen." *Erfahrungsheilkunde,* 1971; 1: 18."

110   Ryan, R.E. "A double–blind clinical evaluation of bromelain in the treatment of acute sinusitis." *Headache,* 1967; 7: 13.

111   Wohlrab, R. "Enzymkombinationspräparat zur therapie der sinusi- tis acuta." *Der Allgemeinarzt,* 1993; 15: 104–114.

112   Barsom, S., Sasse–Rollenhagen, K., Bettermann, A. "Erfolgreiche prostatitisbehandlung mit hydrolytischen enzymen." *Erfahrungsheilkunde,* 1982; 31: 2.

113   Rugendorff, E.W., et al. "Behandlung der chronischen abakteriellen prostatitis mit hydrolytischen enzymen." *Der Kassenarzt,* 1986; 14: 43.

114   Barsom, S., Sasse–Rollenhagen, K., Bettermann, A. "Erfolgreiche prostatitisbehandlung mit hydrolytischen enzymen." *Erfahrungsheilkunde,* 1982; 31: 2.

115   Riede, N.U., et al. *Allgemeine und Spezielle Pathologie.* Stuttgart: Thieme Verlag, 1989.

116   Barsom, S., Sasse–Rollenhagen, K., Bettermann, A. "Zur behandlung von zystitiden und zystopyelitiden mit hydrolytischen enzymen." *Acta Medica Empirica,* 1983; 32: 125.

117   Dittmar, F.–W. & Weisssenbacher, E.R. "Therapie der adnexitis– unterstützung der antibiotischen basisbehandlung durch hydrolytische enzyme." *International Journal of Experimenta and Clinical Chemotherapy,* 1992; 5: 73–82.

118   Pecher, O. *Enzymes: A Drug of the Future.* Ecomed, 1998, pp. 92–95.

119   Griffith, R.S., et al. "Success of L–lysine therapy in frequently recur- rent herpes simplex infection." *Dermatologica,* 1987; 175: 183–190.

120 Kagan, C. "Lysine therapy for herpes simplex." *The Lancet*, 1974; 1:137.

121 Griffith, R., et al. "Relation of arginine–lysine antagonism to herpes simplex growth in tissue culture." *Chemotherapy* 1981; 27: 209–213.

122 Chappa–Alvarez, R. "Pankreatitisbehandlung mit Wobenzym®." Publication in preparation.

123 Sukhikh, G.T., et al. "The therapeutic action of Wobenzym® in multidrug therapy of genitourinary, Chlamydial and mycoplasmal infections." *Oral Enzyme Therapy. Compendium of results from Clinical Studies with Oral Enzyme Therapy. Second Russian Symposium, St. Petersburg, Russia.* Stockdort, Germany: Forum–Medizin, 1997: 39–44.

124 Neuhofer, Ch., et al. "Pathogenetic immune complexes in MS: their elimination by hydrolytic enzymes. A therapeutic approach." International Multiple Sclerosis Conference, Rome, 1988, Monduzzi Editore S.p.A., Bologna.

125 Neuhofer, Ch. "Enzymtherapie bei multipler sklerose." *Hufeland Journal*, 1986; 47.

126 Neuhofer, Ch. "Systemische enzymtherapie bei encephalomyelitis disseminata." *Der prakt Arzt*, 1991; 702.

127 Wrba, H. & Pecher, O. *Enzymes. Medicine of the Future.* Ecomed, 1997, pp. 113–124.

128 Shamburgh, G.E., Jr. "Zinc: an essential trace element." *Clinical Ecology*, 1984; 2(4): 203–206.

129 Scheef, W. "Gutartige veränderungen der weiblichen brust." *Therapiewoche*, 1985: 5090.

130 Scheef, W. "Neue aspekte in der komplexen behandlung von fortgeschirittenen malignen tumoren." In: *Medizinische Enzym-Forschungsgesellschaft* e.V. (ed.): Systemische Enzymtherapie, 3rd Symposium, Vienna, 1988.

131 Dittmar, F.–W., et al. "Wobenzym® zur behandlung der mastophatie." Publication in preparation.

Index

About the Author

Michael W. Loes, M.D., M.D.(H.)

Michael W. Loes, M.D., M.D.(H.) is the director of pain management at Sierra Tucson Hospital. He is a monthly columnist and section editor of *Alternative/Complementary Health and Arthritis* for The National Pain Foundation. He serves as a consultant at Southwest Pain Management and is an assistant professor at the University of Arizona. Dr. Loes has had extensive training in complementary or alternative (integrative) medicine including hypnosis, acupuncture and homeopathy. He serves on a variety of committees and editorial boards and is published extensively.

He has authored and co-authored numerous books, including: *Arthritis: The Doctor's Cure*, *The Aspirin Alternative*, *Healing Sports Injuries Naturally* and *The Healing Power of Jerusalem Artichoke Fiber*, each book exploring the alternative or complementary methods of healing naturally. Dr. Loes recently wrote and published *The Healing Response: Applying the Ten Principles and Laws of Healing*.

He earned his bachelor's degree in linguistics from the University of California at Berkeley and his medical degree from the University of Minnesota Medical School. Dr. Loes completed his internal medicine residency with fellowship training in clinical pharmacology at the University of Arizona and earned further board certifications in addiction and pain medicine. Dr. Loes is certified by boards or qualifying exams in Internal Medicine, Pain Medicine, Pain Management, Alcohol and Chemical Dependency, Acupuncture, Clinical Hypnosis. Homeopathy and Disability Medicine.

Dr. Loes is a popular national speaker addressing strategies to turn on the body's healing response.